COMMUNICATION AND LIVING

COMMUNICATION AND LIVING

Through Time

William J. Russell

To order additional copies of this book, contact:
Xlibris LLC
1-888-795-4274
www.Xlibris.com
Orders@Xlibris.com
611129

Dedication

To Joanne, without your help and gentle pushing,
I would not have completed this work.

This work is dedicated to the collective intellect of all that shall
follow, founded on the knowledge of the past made relevant by
the discoveries of today; especially,
to those who wander in mental quandaries.

And, finally to those who work in the field of
mental health.

PREFACE

(To the first edition)

"We are what we repeatedly do. Excellence, then, is not an act, but a habit."

—Aristotle

For many years, I have carried the baggage that pointed to who I was. I was a son, a father, a soldier; but first, I have always been what I do. Perhaps being a man may have something to do with it, I wonder. Do you wonder too? That is what this book is about, about who you are. Better yet, about who you are as seen by what you do. I often wonder if it is some genetic factor that makes me this or that way, especially, as it pertains to that which I choose to do, my job, my work, my livelihood. Is there some inherent, unseen pressure that makes me choose my livelihood? I believe in Nature/Nurture theory to some degree, but I feel that that "I" am a determining factor too. I believe that I have volition. I have the ability to choose what I am to become. To this end I shall present documentation, material, and other such stuff that you can disagree with, argue with, or point out, "I knew that." Whatever the case, I hope that you will continue to read beyond this point.

In the next several chapters, I shall tackle the job of explaining my point of view by describing the many ways I have been in this world. It may only be a survey of my past, but it may also be a psychological exploration of self-guided by who I have been during each point of contact, with reality as seen by job reference. For some, this may be a way at looking at how job search is performed. For others, it may be a description that defies understanding. At any rate, I hope to explore the self-concept under the microscope of duty. However you define duty, to me, it is the job that I am doing at the present time; further, it may be what I become, my identity, at least momentarily. What must be decided here, in the process of duty, do I become what I do. Moreover, if so, how does that effect who I am? Do we all become what we do? Is the inherent danger that with a loss of what we do create a nonperson? If so, does this nonperson then become an endangered species? Does life then become less important? Is this a time in life that more suicide happens? Or, is this a time in life that merely produces more depression? Some say that if you take away what a man does, you rob him of his identity. If this is true there is certainly much to explore. Let us then, be on our way.

PREFACE

(To the second edition)

"Choose a job you love, and you will never have to work a day in your life."

—Confucius

Although the title, What I Do, seemed like a good one, it did not tell the story correctly. That the emphasis on what a man does is certainly germane, it leaves out the significance of the communication process. Chapter five starts with the hierarchy of learning titled: Communication and Living. Although the focus shall be on what I do, it should carry awareness of the process of communication at all levels. This is especially true as one speaks to self, the non-schizophrenic voice within one's mind that assists with keeping one in touch with reality. The chapters are about the same; changes necessary to understanding and grammar are included.

After reading each chapter, you should contemplate how the information relates to self-communication and to your values about life. The many theoretical approaches that I have made only give clue to my introspection, not to how the world is. Each one must draw their own conclusions. As to validity, truth and goodness, the jury may still be out.

CHAPTER ONE

"Your beliefs don't make you a better person, your behavior does."

—Unknown

PRIMARY IDENTITY

In all that man must feel,
And in all that man must do.
It must certainly be true
That he binds the two,
The feeling and the deed,
Together with his word,
And so perpetuates himself
With myth and seed,
Until he has met his organic
End indeed.
But this end is only
The beginning,
For his myth and seed
Will carry on the deed.[1]

According to Freudian psychology, you begin life, and then you are molded by the many events that occur. Relationships with those around you build your character, personality, and seed your motivation to become. It might be that Freud

---

[1] From The Seduction of Time et al, Xlibris, 2004

gave too much credence to the sexual aspect. I wonder. Sex is important. Is it possible that underlying sexual urges actually create patterns for behavior? The other question one could ask may refer to pathologic states of being. We often have been shown these in detail on TV or in movies. I do not argue that these events do not take place, but rather if they are a primary need for evaluation at this point in my discussion. I choose to look at the healthy aspects of the sex drive at this point. A little later, I may refer to personalities gone astray; especially, from the viewpoint that may be considered sexual, or driven by a sexual impulse. For now, let us deal with the beginning of our persona from the standpoint of normalcy. It is important that we make this distinction early. We need not be concerned with personality aberrations unless they create harm to self or others. We all have minor quirks, and sometimes, it is the very nature of these quirks that create genius.

To start with, I must review what I remember about my first ten years of life. And more importantly, when I first realized that *to do* was important. I grew up in the forties. It was a post war economy and most of the influences of the Second World War could still be seen in the movies. My center of focus, as I played with other kids, was pretending to be at war. To build machine guns out of 2 by 4s, tanks out of cardboard boxes, and create scenes of conflict. After a hard day of playing war though, everyone was able to go home; no one was hurt, it seemed like fun. By the time I was ten years old we had moved to a town in northern California, Willits. Initially, we lived about thirteen or fourteen miles up a road called Sherwood. Back then, I used to get carsick. What fun that was. Each morning on the way to school, it was only a guess whether I would lose my breakfast, or not. It was interesting, for on the way home at night I did not usually get sick. Often this was also, in the winter, a time of day when it was dark, sometimes before we left Willits. My father had an appliance store. I often got to play in the back of the store. It was musty and had dirt on one end. There were many black widow spiders as well. After school, I would always hang around until it was time to go on the long ride home. How I dreaded that ride. Everything was peaceful. No war, no bad times, and school were, well, all right.

I was always a dreamer. I could sit right in front of you, appear to be listening, but be miles away. I think that even today I am able to do that at great annoyance to anyone talking to me. I have a problem with thinking. You see, I am able to think so fast that I have unused time when listening. Often I try to assist the person talking with their thoughts. This too creates discourse. It is most often embarrassing when I interrupt someone trying to fill-in what they say, only to find out that I was completely wrong with my assessment. I am sure that this alienates many, who might otherwise choose to be my friend. My father would often remind that I should spend more time doing chores around the house.

After about one year living up Sherwood road, my family bought a house about one mile from town on the same road. Along with this great house, we also had about seventy-five acres. This was a good time in my life. At some point, I had gotten interested in chemistry. Unfortunately, my big emphasis was in how to make a bomb. With seventy-five acres to explore,

I was able to set off quite a few tests without ever being noticed. I think that because someone was always detonating dynamite, I was not found out, at least not in the first years. When I later decided to sell bombs that was when I was really noticed, especially when in school. I had a friend one who bought one of my products and set it off in the schoolyard. He was out in the baseball bleachers. When he set the bomb off it flew over and supposedly hit a steam engine about a quarter of mile away. Naturally, the school principle got a call. And naturally, the person setting off the bomb was called in to the office. And most naturally, of all, he gave me up to the principle. I met the principle with my father that same day. I was told to start a new hobby, photography. That Christmas I got some real neat stuff for photography. However, before that, I was told to get rid of all my explosive products. My dad was to inspect my lab. He would determine if I had done what they had requested. I remember this with a smile. He did not have any idea what was or was not explosive, or could be used to create explosions. He came up to my room. Looked over what I had, smiled and said, "OK son" and left. I don't think that he noticed the sulfuric acid, about nine pounds, the powdered magnesium, the potassium chlorate, or sulfur, or ammonium nitrate. It just was not his thing, and I knew that. He was one hell of a mechanic. Like Clint Eastwood said, "Every man has got to know is limitation." Although I did take up photography, I really did not ever stop with the bombs. I just became much more careful.

There is always a second time. I had a friend stay overnight once. It seems that he was most interested in my experiments with ammonium nitrate, zinc, and glycerin. Unbelievably, this guy was sitting in front of me during one of my classes, and he literally blew up. There was a blinding flash (no he did not change into captain marvel), and his shirt was on fire. He ran to the front of the room and the teacher, an older woman, ripped his shirt off and stomped on it. There was no damage to him, her, or the room. Well, other than all I could see was an after flash indelibly imprinted in my brain, one that took several hours to go away, I was no worse for the incident, at least not physically. Therefore, off to the principle he went. You guessed it. He told the principle that I had sold him the stuff. I do not remember selling him the stuff, but it seems logical, to me, that I would not have sold him a bomb that would explode in his pocket. In addition, I do not believe he had the smarts to build one. At any rate, I met the principle with my father. It was not so peaceful this time. I had a few days to think about this. In addition, I was given a few jobs around the house and had to help my father on weekends. He was building a dress shop for my mother. A house had burned in Willits. Evidently, my Dad had been given permission to salvage the bricks from the fireplace. It was my job, on Saturday, to clean off every brick and stack them so that he could pick them up after work. I thought that my world had ended. It was time for some restructuring of the *who* in *who I was*. Perhaps photography was not so bad after all.

Living on a ranch was fun. My mother, my dad and I each had a horse to ride. I had gotten my first horse when I was twelve years old. His name was sleepy. He was a retired cattle horse. He taught me a lot. By the time we moved down to the new house one mile from town, sleepy was gone or sold, I do not remember. On the new ranch, we had three horses. One called playboy. He was a gilding 16 plus hands tall and smart as a whip. He once saved my dad's life. The story goes that my dad was hunting up in Modoc county California. He was astride playboy on a steep path. It was narrow and the fall beneath quite long. There was barely room for horse and man. They came to where a tree had fallen down hill and stuck on the path. Someone had cut the tree a bit allowing room to walk through. Playboy started to go over it, but as he did, the log began to slide. Playboy reared up on his hindquarters and turned completely in the direction from which they came, then, carefully lowered his forequarters until it was again safe. The log crashed below. Playboy shivered. My dad got off and led him back to a safe place, and neither my dad nor playboy ever mentioned it again; well, except to tell me so that I could tell you.

My dad was an excellent mechanic, outdoorsman, and philosopher. He often would give me examples of how something should be. And, often it was not so. That is, it should have been, but it just was not. He spoke of a job well done. He related that one should do a day's labor for a day's pay, and that any job worth doing was worth doing right. A man was his word. Moreover, a John Wayne style of dispersing what was right had gotten him into many fights when he was young. I remember when I was only about four or five in Chicago how he defended what he felt was right. We were in a restaurant eating. My mother was a beautiful redhead. Two men dressed in pin stripe suits were sitting not too far away from us. Evidently, one man made a remark about my mother. My dad got up and calmly walked over to them. He leaned over and said something to them. One of them made a remark. At that point, he grabbed both of them by their collars and bounced their heads together. They slid placidly to the floor. A waiter came and asked my father if there was a problem, and he mentioned that the two men should not be sleeping, but rather be eating. The waiter looked over at them, smiled and had them escorted out of the restaurant. One can only think about the possibilities those days. They both may have been packing, God knows. But my father, like John Wayne, was a man of few words when it came to things like that. He was fiercely strong, and I doubt that he feared anyone. His persona often put him in peril. His rush against time eventuated in him dying of a massive coronary thrombosis at the age of fifty-two.

Well into my second decade, I had established some strong beliefs about what a man was. However, I had not yet established what I was to become. The problem with growing up as I did, in those times, was that I had it so good that I did not have to worry, let alone create any self-motivation. My parents often pushed me to get a job, do something! I did not have a clue. I was not mature enough, even at fifteen. I did not graduate from high school until I was nineteen. I was drafted at twenty-one.

At twenty-one most of the self-communication, for me, was not from me. I began to realize that I was allowing others to tell me, influence me, and to form opinions that I would later reject. Maturation is learning to separate self from others when it comes to evaluations about how the world is. Belief systems are built from these communications with self. Evaluation of life, like this writing, is part of this process; reflection brings closure.

CHAPTER TWO

FIRST HINT

It was my dream to go to college. However, I did not do that well in high school, and by the time I realized that it would have been a good idea to have As and Bs, I was a junior, and that, my friend is too late for any kind of scholarship. As an idealistic dreamer, I had wandered my way through the most important years of living without really paying attention. No matter how much you tell your children, you cannot change them by only talking to them. Worst of all, you cannot change them by yelling at them. My parents had a bad habit of not doing anything until I was in deep stuff; then, the yelling began. It was not helpful.

So I am out of high school. I am nineteen. I have no job, although I have done a few things, nothing steady. I decide to go to Santa Rosa Junior College. My parents are willing to help me, but I really need to find work while I am there. With my thinking, that chemistry would be great, because I know all about bombs, I sign up for a major in chemistry. Boy was that a mistake. First off, my math skills are dreary at best. We did not have computers to do everything for us in 1953. Moreover, I did not take enough credits to be exempt from the draft. When I started failing some of my classes that was not good either. Sometime in 1953, I got a draft call. I reported to the induction center.

It was one horrendous experience. Picture a large number of men clad only in their underwear. We stood in long lines. At one point, we were all seated, probably about ten or so, to have blood taken. Along comes a corpsman dressed in white. He has tubes and sterile needles. He gives you a tube, and asks you to hold it. He sticks a needle in your arm and tells you to hold the tube under the needle and allow blood to run into it, oh yeah, yell when it is full. My thinking is if you didn't pass out your a marine, just a little dizzy, the army, and on the floor, the air force. Or not.

At one point, we had x-rays taken if we had given them a reason to do so. I had an old injury to my right ankle while tumbling in college. What the heck, they might find something, so I complained of pain in my ankle and foot. Low and behold, the x-ray showed a nonunion fracture in my right big toe. Evidently, they did not want to take a chance that this may interfere with basic training and I was given my freedom. However, it was to be short-lived. In six months I was to report again, this time I was not so lucky.

On May 14 1954, I was inducted into the United States Army and proceeded to Fort Ord, California. I was not alone, as a friend of mine, Jimmy Borders, had gotten the call too. We went together. I will never forget that first night in the barracks, sleeping amongst all those other young men. Bunk beds full of farting, snoring scared young men. The smell of the new bedding, clothes, and army gear still permeates my brain today, fifty-nine years later.[2] I was an only child. Being with others was something new to me. Nevertheless, in time, I became close to

---

[2]   As of this rewrite date January 2014.

many of the men and we enjoyed a kind of camaraderie that I had not known before. As a child, I had always been a loner, staying to myself and doing things my way. In the army there were three ways to do things, the right way, the wrong way, and the army way. We did it the army way. Unfortunately, I did not finish basic with my new friends or Jim. About four weeks into basic, I got pneumonia. I was hospitalized and that was the cause for me to lose my company. I never saw Jimmy Borders again in those first two years. After getting back to another basic training company, I graduated. I received orders to attend the Quarter Master School, Fort Lee, Virginia. From there I came back to Fort Ord and finished a very uneventful first two years in the service of my country.

One bright sun shiny day in May, two years to the day from my induction, I was once again to become a civilian. Oh happy day I thought. Now I could get back to doing the things that I considered important. I still did not have a hint of what I would become, or even what I wanted to do in my life. Returning back to Willits was a little like returning to the past where I had left off. My grades at Santa Rosa Junior College were barely good enough for me to go to another school. My parents had completely redone my room. In my pocket, I had only one hundred dollars of mustering-out pay from the army. In addition, there was no job in sight. The summer of 1956 was a poor time to find work and 1957 was not going to be any better. But, as luck would have it, there was a job opening with the Pacific Gas and Electric Company in Willits. It was a job working with a unit that repaired pipes, digging ditches, and everything required to keep the water flowing, both ways. I got one heck of a suntan and developed some great muscles from the hard labor. It was not my forte, but it paid a fair wage. My parents decided to charge me fifty dollars a month for room and board. It seemed fair to me and things were really quite pleasant. I had a job, a little money, and time to myself when I needed it. However, I still did not have a hint. One day a fellow classmate from high school who was working in the office as a meter book clerk decided to quit. During lunchtime, I got a note to report to the office. I was interviewed by the district manager and within days found myself working as a meter book clerk with little training. Single entry book keeping was not new to me; I had been a supply clerk in the army. I knew something about paperwork. It was actually quite an interesting job. My responsibilities were many, but the main duty was making entries into books that were sent out to be tabulated for billing. So, if I made an error it would show up on the client's bill. Usually any error had to do with an entry of numbers into the books from the tags turned in by the meter readers. I made a few. In addition, there were the usual over readings and the like. I also had a money drawer. I had thirty dollars in that drawer. I remember once on payday that I had borrowed some money from my drawer to buy lunch. My thinking was who would know, as soon as I cashed my check, I would put it back. Not right, while I was out to lunch a co-worker decided to balance my drawer for me. Right, I came up short. When I got back, there was a note that I had to speak with the assistant manager. In a calm voice, he began with the time of day, the weather, and finally got down to what was troubling him. I told the truth. I am not sure that he believed me to this day. A notation made in my personnel record and that was it. The following year I returned to college.

Chico State College was a vastly new experience. Moreover, even at 24 I still do not think that I had a clue. By this time, I had decided that psychology would be a good major. Chemistry had been a disaster. I had gotten to Chico in the summer months before school. I had the G.I. bill at about $110.00 per month, but no job. Therefore, I took odd jobs to try to build up some money to add to the $500.00 I had saved from the P, G, &E. By the time school started, I had gotten my first G.I. check, but still had no steady work. I rented a room in a big house. I was on the second floor with access to a great bathroom. My rent was $50.00 each month. My meals averaged about $10.00 each day, or so. Now I have roughly $60.00 left for books and whatever. Even back in 1957, $60.00 was not that much. By the time, I had registered for my first class I had dipped well into my $500.00 reserve. I had to find a job.

They call it serendipity, in one of my classes I ran into a young man named Bob. It so happened that his uncle had, or more than likely, operated a grocery store in Chico. Bob told me that I should go down and see if he needed help. Bob was almost sure that Ernie needed someone to stock shelves. I did, and I got the job. It was minimum wage, but it was steady work. Now I was better able to concentrate on school.

My first year at Chico was a time for a beginning hint. I think that I had an inkling of what my life direction was to become. Psychology was a good major, but I had other subjects that were required. I also took a course in public speaking. My very first time in front of an audience was something like the Don Knotts portrayal that I had seen on TV once. Stage fright almost immobilized me to the point of catatonia. I made it through that first time. I learned to recognize that stage fright was, for me, really just an adrenalin rush created by my intense desire to speak, to act, to be the center point of attention. Although it would be several years before I got real control of this rush, in the end I believe that I learned to use it in a way to assist me with what I would eventually do best. It was truly a beginning. Speaking is not enough; one has to have a focus.

Along with an introduction courses in psychology, I was required to take an English course and one having to do with writing. Part of the writing concerned poetry. Not only did we have to read poetry in the text, but we were encouraged to write some as well. In 1957, poetry, for men, especially during this time of John Wayne, was not of primary emphasis. While I do not think it was a sissy thing to do, it was not something that was encouraged outside of creative writing classes in those days. Following is one of the first poems that I wrote.

I Am What I Am

I am a very definite me,
And perhaps, you are a very definite you.
Probably, there is no other way to be,
To be someone else, a hard thing to do;
And, the same holds true for me.
Even though I try, I try in vain,

I find that in the end I am myself,
And with you it must be the same.
We are both stuck with a certain
                Inescapable self,
All bound and tagged with a specific name.
It is hard to say which factor decides the real you.
The name or you per se.
Or, there might still be another factor too,
One that makes you this or that way.
But when all is said and done,
We find that we are no more than we,
A bit of seriousness and a bit of pun.
After all what else is there for us to be,
But, ourselves, for what is done, is done.[3]

This may be a first glimpse of my limited insight into who I was to become, more than a hint, less than a persona. There were several other poems written that year, but none that I considered earth shaking. I was finding myself. I only completed one year at Chico, my next endeavor was to be more than twenty years.

---

[3]   The Seduction of Time et al, W.J. Russell, Xlibris, 2004, pg 57

CHAPTER THREE

A STERN REALITY

June 1958 was beginning of many things, but foremost among them was my marriage to a Willits girl and my reentrance to the military. The plan was, even though a few days before my marriage, that I would be enlisted as married. This reduced adding to the confusion in later paperwork. The paperwork done, I had one week to be married and report for induction. The honeymoon was short, and I felt like I was going back to something that I was not sure. Doubt clouded my mind and probably spoiled what should have been a joyous time in my young life. I was 25 and my wife only 17. Although I would like to spend a little time about our marriage, that is not the focus of this work. The first twenty years of marriage was a happy time in my life and we brought into the world four sons, all born in military hospitals; One in Japan.

I was told that I would have to take a test and then probably would not have to take basic training all over again. Right, no such thing happened. I took the battery of tests, did not pass go, but went directly to a training company at good old Fort Ord. I must admit though, it was much easier the second time. After basic, I was ordered to Brooke Army Medical Center Fort Sam Houston, Texas to attend a basic course in neuropsychiatric procedures. This had something to do with the fact that I had attended Chico State and had stated that my major was psychology. I had also shown a proclivity to psychology on the induction tests. I think that one of the tests was a personality survey. Therefore, I was on my way to Fort Sam.

There is always one more thing, you know, like Colombo. Before I could take the neuropsychiatric theory, I had to take basic medical training followed by four weeks of neuropsychiatric classroom training. Most of the theory, laden heavily with Freudian constructs. One psychiatrist, an older man in his fifties, babbled on about how most schizoid personalities and schizophrenics were latent homosexuals. That homosexuality was an aberration of pathological proportions, ad infinitum. A psychiatric nurse spoke to us as well. Her basic concern had to do with working on the ward with the mentally ill. This was to be our future as neuropsychiatric specialists. Moreover, the information that she imparted still rings true today. She was a most humane person, caring, understanding and nonjudgmental. The mentally ill were only different in a matter of degree, she had stated. It was to this degree that we would apply our new learned skills. A major emphasis, back then, was to prevent suicide. Often the psychiatric wards were full and many were suicidal.

After four weeks of neuropsychiatric training, orders were cut for our next assignment. Mine was at Letterman General Hospital, presidio of San Francisco, California. I began my married life, my career in the army, and my journey into self January 1959. I was soon to be 26 years old. It was at this time in my life that I discovered writing. One of my first works had to do with an exploration of the three basic structures of the human personality. I called them, the psychespiritual, psychochemical, and psychointellectual orientations to organic[4] reality. It was esoteric stuff back then. I wrote over 125 pages of theoretical implications having to do with this subject in a book with the title, "An Introduction into Moral Psychology." I still have the writings today. What was once possibly shocking is now mundane. We have come so far that what I once believed to be theoretical has now become naked reality. At least, much of the controversy has been, cussed and discussed ad nauseam. An example follows. Brought up to date, to a degree, but the basic intent and philosophy still pervades the writing.

BEYOND OEDIPUS
A PROBLEM WITH IDENTIFICATION
(Communication from the unconscious)

Any theory of personality must certainly be a search for self. In fact, such an endeavor to uncover any inherent truth about personality must admit to the ubiquitously absurd nature of such a task; for, it is obvious that not one being is ever like another. What instead must follow, is the conclusion that there must exist similarities in the nature of the human mind, that our experience and therefore our behaviors are the consequence of natural laws, that our minds, and therefore the byproducts of our minds existence, personality, are part of the matter from which we are made, a proprioceptive[5] truth that needs verification with contact from an outside reality.

---

4   Organic, as in life.
5   The process of receiving stimuli within the tissues of the body; as within muscles and tendons.

In every theory there exists a moment of thought that seems to be the cornerstone of its existence. In the Freudian personality theory, I identify this cornerstone as being the Oedipus complex and myth.

The Oedipus Myth in Retrospect

The myth seems to be a fundamental aspect within Freudian thought, laden heavily with incestuous implications, and fraught with the concomitants of such relationships. Kin Oedipus is destined to kill his Father and have sex with his Mother; this seems evident even before his birth (predicted by an oracle of Jocasta's enwombed child). It is a punctuation of the event in time, considered in the here-and-now, by language connotations that may implicate different meanings today. A myth is still a myth, perhaps not a reality at all.

The story is that Laius, king of Thebes, was warned by an oracle that his son would slay him. Accordingly when his wife, Iocaste (in Homer Epicaste), bore a son, she exposed the baby on Mt. Cithaeron, first pinning his ankles together, hence the name Oedipus, "swell-foot" in order to ensure that no one would save the child, if found, or perhaps to make it impossible for his ghost to walk. A Corinthian shepherd took pity on the infant, who was adopted by the childless Polybus, King of Corinth, and his wife, and brought up as their son. In early manhood, Oedipus was taunted by a drunkard, concerning his parentage, and he visited Delphi to learn the truth. The oracle informed him that he was fated to kill his father and marry his mother, so he resolved never to return to Corinth.

Traveling toward Thebes, he encountered Laius, who provoked a quarrel in which Oedipus killed him. Continuing on his way, Oedipus found Thebes plagued by the sphinx, a fabulous winged monster, half-human, half-leonine, who put a riddle to all passersby and destroyed those who could not answer. Oedipus solved the riddle[6], and the sphinx killed herself. In reward, he received the throne of Thebes and the hand of the widow queen, his mother, Iocaste. They had four children: Eteocles, Polynices, Antigone, and Ismene. Subsequently the whole truth became known. Iocaste committed suicide, and Oedipus, after blinding himself, shunned the daylight in the palace, or (in Sophocles' version) went into exile, accompanied by Antigone and Ismene, leaving his brother-in-law Creon as regent. He met his end at Colonus near Athens, where he was swallowed into the earth and became a guardian hero of the land. One might say swallowed into the *bowels* of the earth, a possible double meaning or a play on the word with Colonus.

The myth is complex and may be laden with semantic quandaries, ones that speak beyond the story in an abstraction far above any concrete reference that we can make today. The time is gone, and so too are the players, far from the organic, wisps of air leaving their traces in the words of the myth recreated by different personalities, and used by others for their end. So when I think of Freud, it must be that he used the myth as an example, it could no more be factual than could the creature named sphinx. If this is true, then I am able to speak to

---

[6] The riddle—"What is it which first goes on four, then on two, and eventually on three?" The answer, "Man." First as a child on all four, then as a man on two, and finally with a cane.

the words used and about their relationship to each other. When you play with a metaphor, do so at your own risk, but at the very least, do so with the *present day* in mind. Language should always be brought up to date without losing meanings from the past, as past meanings color our present.

Although there is much mention of the relationship between father and son in the myth, it seems that the focus should be the one between Oedipus and his mother Iocaste. In his book, *The Forgotten Language*, Erich Fromm raises the issue of incest, "we have raised the question whether, if incest was the essence of Oedipus's crime, the drama should have told us that he had fallen in love with Jocasta unwittingly." In *Oedipus at Colonus*, Sophocles has Oedipus himself answer this question when he states, "Thebes bound me, unknowingly, to the bride that was my curse." The marriage to her was not the outcome of his own *desire*, and decision, instead, she was one of the rewards for the city's savior.

The foregoing does a very good job of separating love from desire symbolically. I am sure that Jocasta did not force Oedipus to copulate with her. Indeed, there must have been something that called forth the force between his loins. I submit that this symbolic representation calls upon us to look closer at this aspect of the Oedipus myth.

It is not until Jocasta gives birth to children by her son that problems arise. If we focus on this part of their relationship, we may find some interesting symbolic language that speaks to us today, perhaps into eternity as well.

Late Oedipus complex

During the early years, a young boy must transfer his feelings of a sexual nature from his mother to another female, a process usually culminating in sexual union or marriage, and thereafter the process seems to be a cooling one from the standpoint of sexual desire. Early Oedipal fixations become subliminal, but retain their ability to come to consciousness in an altered form. As in the myth, as soon as the wife becomes a mother the repressed symbol fixation is unearthed with a new identity focus. The wife becomes a mother. The symbol mother and the actuality of motherhood physiologically fuse into one. Now it is difficult to feel sexual desire towards this new object. The wife becomes the *old lady*, the giver of milk and honey. So strong is this identification (subliminally) process that you may find some men cheating on their wife sexually, but still claiming to love her. A kind of divided loyalty exists between desire and love without desire. Here, as in the myth, love has been split from desire. Where sexual gratification has been identified as *dirty* in childhood, and all the words used to describe its glory, you will find overt behavior pitting its strength against these feelings and words being felt and being used in the presence of the nurturing mother. The late Oedipus complex is now complete, full-blown and spreading its self. The man has again a mother to care for his split libidinous self, a chasm that may last for the rest of his life.

The idea of a *late reverse Oedipus complex* creates another direction for treatment of personality dysfunction. It would seem logical to investigate this aspect both in the child and in the adult. In the past, the task was difficult because it was believed that some change might have taken place in the personality. Rather than change, it would seem that the process is one of continuation, where the late reverse complex reveals itself in adulthood.

A problem that one encounters regarding the reverse Oedipus personality concept is in the situation where a cheating man has relations with another married woman with children. This would lead one to believe that cheating was certainly different in this situation from the cheating created by a late reverse Oedipus complex. Perhaps there is much more to this aspect of personality than we could ever imagine. What we must conclude is that while a late Oedipus complex certainly is possible, its existence or nonexistence will do little to give us total understanding about the cheating aspect of men in the situation of coercive marriage. Therefore, I must infer that cheating by itself, does neither prove nor disprove the existence of a late reverse Oedipus complex.

Long-term relationships within a marriage seem best fitted to encourage the development of a late Oedipus response. When the male is passing the forty-year mark and the marriage has lasted half this time a predisposition for this behavior may have been generated. Some would call this a last fling, unfinished business, or a second childhood. What it may be is a return to the touch of youth, semantically stating to yourself that you feel younger every day. Especially if you mean by feeling young to touch someone young, to unite with another polarity in orgasm momentarily *becoming* with that person where all evidence of self is set aside, or merging your identity with the other self.

Whether or not this oneness with another could be considered late Oedipus or the quest for lost youth is difficult to determine. Sexuality has a symbolic relationship with immortality, and somewhere within this relationship, the concept of youth must certainly reside.

The foregoing has done little to confirm the existence of a late reverse Oedipus personality disorder, but I believe it may have created a question or two. What is it that seems to draw men into these kinds of relationships when they appear to be happily married? Better yet, in the light of the complexity of the marriage situation what is it that keeps men from going astray sexually? Is it love? Love is a term describing a physiological relationship between two organisms that lasts but 20-30 seconds involuntarily controlled by endocrine and/ or pheromone response, all else subsumed under the rubric of companionship. If love is the cohesive force that holds marriage together, the preceding may create some anxiety in those holding this belief. It would be more considerate to say that love was the starting point from which a relationship either did or did not develop. Furthermore, that when this relationship involved a young single female with an older married man, that it is described in terms of the concept of late reverse Oedipus personality behavior. With this statement, we have a way to describe the defined behavior in terms of the Oedipus complex, but in a more specific way. Since we have identified sexuality as a core problem and have shown that the Oedipus myth has split love from sexual desire, it may be important to discuss love and sexuality.

Meaning Point

The process of communicating with self may be evident. In a Freudian way, the late Oedipus complex is nothing more than communication that may be subconscious regarding the process of identification of the wife as *the mother,* rather than *a mother.*

Moreover, it is this unconscious feeling that points to incest.

Love, a Unique Problem of Being

Is love a term describing a physiological relationship between two organisms that lasts but 20 to 30 seconds, involuntarily controlled by endocrine and/or pheromone response, while all else may be subsumed under the rubric of companionship?

The foregoing precise definition of love as a psychochemical response most certainly leaves out the emotional aspect as well as the spiritual involvement within the ego boundaries during the pre-exciting, orgasmic, and post-rest phase of sexual activity.

Only a fool would deny the inner existence of a profound feeling for another when both spirit (psyche) and body meld. It is this unmelding which creates a feeling vacuum when this touch is lost, the very separation painful to the core of the personalities so entwined; albeit, there are times that only one may be grossly affected, but no one can doubt that something has taken place at the unconscious level of being. For one brief moment, two souls have touched in primal fusion.[7]

Sexual love is a special kind of touch. It is the ultimate of nonverbal communication, where two polarities fuse together to momentarily become one; ego boundaries shedding their outer capsules and briefly harmonizing to the human container's rhythmic throes. This cadence transcends time and flesh and hastens to the call of immortality. However, to soon this touch recedes leaving an emotional backwash that may incur the sweet pain of separation. The nectar of love acts as a narcotic to the emotional substance of being that is most addicting. This archaic need reaching out of the grave of time speaking to all who must travel this road making contact in the form of primal fusion, never again to be the same, never again totally alone. As in the last stanza of the poem Ecstasy[8]

Sweet daggers passion dipped,[9]
Into entrails embedded,
Tasting nectar of love composed;
Two chemistries entwined,
Exploding, mixing timeless souls.

Emotional love rides on the wave of heated passion, for the mind must always obey the body, imprisoned in this burning now. Ego boundaries cling to the reality that the personality serves up, often consumed by vast emotional surges that lash

---

7   A term used in the book, Meaning the love of one sex cell for another; *The Sexual Life of Our Time*, Bloch, Iwan, MD, Allied Book Company, NY, 1928.

8   The Seduction of Time, et al, William J. Russell, Xlibris, 2004.

9   Also, the ending poem in the book, *Murder in C-Minor*, Wm. J. Russell, 2007.

deep into the very psyche of being. These tracings cut deep into the core of the personality leaving scars (imprints) for life, ones with feedback propensities beyond this time, often stirred to life by a tune, a smell, a sight, or by purposeful recall. Emotional healing from such lovesick phenomena must take a time that is many times greater than the initial exposure to the sexual object to heal.

Only total loss of ego boundaries without immediate return can be emotionally dangerous. One must assume that partial loss is often the case and may very well be the cause of the emotional pain. In this process of redefining the self one must fit the loved object into the personal self in a way that is in harmony with the system of reference, i.e., give new meaning to the existing ego boundaries; perhaps include the other self within them. Often this process is difficult since the sexual shock of two personalities so entwined make ego identity nebulous at the moment of fusion. A period of 20 or 30 seconds, or a bit more, may not be enough for one to become one with another personality since all parts of the personal self may not be available at the moment of sexual orgasm. Therefore, it must be that although emotional love does begin early during sexual union, true emotional love needs time to grow and many more fusions to blossom entirely on its own.

Emotional love stands the test of time while sexual love may fade as the human container ages and goes into physiological rust, a condition often found in marriage beyond the 30-year mark, although this physiological rust may be more a process of the mind rather than the body. If the emotional component

Russell

is made strong, it is theoretically possible for the love condition to last a lifetime. This may require being able to feel beyond the body container, or it may intimate the actuality of one soul mate for life. It is easy to see that many marriages do not meet the foregoing, as the sexual interest span seems to be tantamount to the life span of the relationship, as in the reverse Oedipus complex.

How would one make love new? Would it take more than mere sexual technique, since the intimation is that fusion is but the spark in the haystack of love? Does sack-time necessarily equate with marriage longevity? Does the body beautiful state of existence as an idea within our culture setting point to a stagnation of emotional love? If any answer to these questions can make itself known, it seems likely that it will indicate a pattern of personality development or change in behavior. It is postulated that the concept of personality contains within its meaning the philosophical relationship between body and mind that make an individual a persistent entity as can be seen by enduring patterns of behavior. Enduring patterns of behavior identify specific personalities. In order to make an assessment about personality one must be able to communicate with the personality in question and with others within the same cultural setting and time. The questions often asked by those concerned, "Is love a special form of communication? Indeed, is love at the core of all forms of communication?" If so, "In what way and how can we use our knowledge about this form of communication to aid in self healing, better understanding, and producing longer life in better health?"

To better understand, or create a pathway to understanding, I have created a communication paradigm.

The Three Spaces

The space of sight gives one the ability to observe another's behavior, while the voice space brings to one how another's voice may sound, and certainly the contact space of touch and olfaction bring one to the acme of understanding. Each space contributes to total understanding until touch/olfaction give rise to the highest form of nonverbal communication. The touch of sexual contact considered here.

At the very outset of time, humankind demonstrated a division, namely two sexes. This suggests several events. The two had no knowledge of sex, and therefore had to learn by touch. They had a given language, and therefore spoke to each other. Someone else told them (the snake), or by Divine intervention. With a combination of nonverbal and verbal communication, they came to the realization of sexual congress. Or, there was a kind of *fusion love*, love of one cell for another, primal gametes. Then from the primal ooze, we sprang.

The idea of primal gametes gives rise to a possible plus or minus relationship indicating that we are in some way chemically attracted to another. This could mean that from the very beginning we have related to one another in a chemical way. As our structure became more complex, love as fusion, became more distant. We are now reacting to a process of sexual congress and fusion with billions of accessory cells no longer directly responsible for the primary fusion of the gametes. This form of sexual love is an abstraction of the gametes fusion, although at the moment of contact between sperm and egg a chemical message sings throughout the body of the female. Much later a child is born.

Love then, in its primary stage is no more than the attraction of a sperm for an ovum, chemical polarity that determines the oncoming age of man, and the process that each new human must pass through to become a new life. The idea of touch is deeply woven into the primal gamete logic. Man must try to touch his reproductive cell with another; this, a form of communication that promises him immortality, this special touch, a communication that beckons to the future and provides intense organic feeling for the present.

The suggestion of polarity describes what sexual communication began as a process of one cell mass attracted to another. Fusion gave new life. In the broadest sense, this is all that there is to the concept of primal fusion. The process also serves as a form of primal communication. Survival of the species is the promise of this communication. Today, in the distant future what has changed? Communication still takes place, but as a kind of distant love. Talk leads to seduction if the climate is right. Some say that distance reduction to the level of touch is all that communication was designed to do. We need no tower of babble today, for the process of communication has become so complex, that at times, we cannot even get a message across to a friend. Nations fight wars based on syntax of confusion, misunderstanding, and verbal dysfunction.

WORDS ARE THINGS

Words are things,
That wars are made from,
And war certainly
Presupposes
The existence of man;
And, mankind speaks
To itself,
One humankind to another,
For it takes more than one
To hold a conversation,
And more than one,
To bust two heads together.

The Valence of Sexuality

If there is such a thing as sexual polarity, as in the foregoing a communication that is primal, and seeks to perpetuate the human model in organic reality, then we should begin with a theoretical model describing how that might be.

Using the magic triad let us suppose that three distinct parts of personality exist, namely; psychochemical, psychointellectual, and psychospiritual. These integrated parts act upon the whole of one persona, and deeply into the sexual being. The psychochemical orientation intends to indicate that which is chemical (pheromone), or perhaps physiological, while the psychointellectual aspect is consonant with the part of the sexual being that is determined by the mind in the various states of consciousness, but primarily the state of awareness. The last part of the triad considers the religious point of view. Although believed by many that the need for God is self evident within the species, it is felt that the true meaning within the psychospiritual orientation (also psychespiritual) comes from outside the mind and is an exogenous process. It is an operating force that keeps humankind a continuing presence in nature and is therefore included as part of the triad. When it becomes necessary to explain an act in the light of the psychospiritual orientation to organic reality, it will have something to do with ones conception of God, religious ideology, or ones belief but dealing with an exogenous force. Even the negation of belief may present with symptoms. To deny God infers His existence.

Some entertain the idea that normal is what is average, that for the most part, normal is dictated by the multitude, and that we can consider any exaggerations as ones coming from unique personalities that might be normal for another culture, group, or place in time. What is outside our average concept is an aberration of personality. Since psychological diagnosis is based upon occurrence and intensity of any particular orientation, we should admit that there is much room for disagreement, especially within the area of personality theory. There are volumes written about personality theory. There is however, a slim thread of evidence holding all theories together, that being in man's unique awareness of self. Awareness of self implies something beyond physical matter. In addition, from this derives a host of theoretical implications. One does not question the passage of time, the existence of self, or finiteness of life. We instead question their properties. So is the case of sexuality and the part it plays in the formation of personality. The triad is another point of view.

In short, psychochemical relates to physiological need, the psychointellectual connotes awareness of that need, and psychospiritual purifies the need by moral reflection. In all, the valence of sexuality is determined by the interacting parts of the personality. When imbalance occurs, or part of the triad is missing there is an aberration in the personality that may lead to a psychological diagnosis.

Having written the foregoing, I tried to get it published. However, I had no funds for such an endeavor, having recently gotten married and a child on the way. My income was a sparse $140.00 each month in the military. Once I won a $10.00 baseball pool, enough to buy food for the last four days of the month. Times were hard in the military, but medical care was good. I was a neuropsychiatric technician. The job was horrendous. We had little else than electroshock therapy and a few drugs to combat the unknown. While the virus of psychiatry, schizophrenia, ran rampant in the halls. We gave huge amounts of Thorazine (compared to today's standards) to those who seemed most out of control. We called it psychosis. Some say today, that perhaps schizophrenia is just another form of communication, pathological, but an attempt to make contact. Others state it as an attempt to rid the body of the demons of an organic nature. It may be a little of both with a great part unknown. I remained in the field of neuropsychiatry for about four years. Late in 1962, I changed my field to orthopaedics. It was a course given at Letterman General Hospital, Presidio of San Francisco. There were just two of us in the training. It was a great change. I had just moved from the abstract field of psychiatry to the concrete field of orthopaedics, from mind to plaster in four months. Now I was again a new person in the light of what I did.

My title was a cast specialist. For the next five years, I worked with plaster, not the wall kind, but the plaster of Paris of healing. I was 29 years old. With the ending of the third decade of life, I was just beginning to get a hint of what I was to become. The search for self is a life journey. Most do not know even at the end of life what they have become let alone know what the "I" is in "what I do." With orthopaedics as a focus, a job, I began to take on an interest in teaching others.

CHAPTER FOUR

THE WORLD OF PLASTER

Things heal faster in plaster. To focus on the concrete was an absolute. It brings you in touch with concrete reality. You do not take your work home with you. You put on a cast. If done correctly, nothing further is needed at that moment. When you work on a mental health ward, it sticks to you like the scent of death. Plaster is pleasant. You mold with your hands. You touch someone in a special way. You assist with physical healing. You can take pride in your work because it is visible. Not all work a cast specialist does is great. Taking off a cast the first time can be a little frightening to the patient and yourself. Eventually you will cut someone with a cast blade. The blade does not rotate; it oscillates about a quarter of an inch at the periphery. This means that if you hold the cast saw correctly, you will probably jiggle the skin below when you get close. If you are cutting over a bone, there is always a chance that you might push too hard and cut the skin. If over a boney prominence, you may even slice the periosteum[10]. This has potential to be an open fracture. If you define a fracture as any break in the continuity of the boney cortex, it is. The time when this is most likely to happen is when you bivalve a wet cast after surgery. This is done to allow for possible swelling and still create immobilization. It happened to me the first time that I made a mono-valve cut in a long leg cast after surgery. After cutting the full length of the wet cast, I

---

[10]   Best to think of this as a kind of bone skin.

spread the cast to find red stuff in the cotton padding—not a good sign. That army ranger probably has a small scar to this day.

After my four months of training, I graduated. I got orders to report to Fort Sill, Oklahoma. It was January 1963; I would be thirty in February. The third decade of life had passed. I was still in the phase of *becoming*, I had not yet realized what I would become, I was, however, not in limbo. With a background in neuropsychiatry, photography, some chemistry, and a familiarity with audiovisual equipment, I would now make my way into the arena of teaching. One needs maturity and education for this challenge. I had a little of both. Some would say not enough. The years to come would prove to be anything but boring. The Army would not let me stagnate; I would be constantly on the move, both in time and in mind. A cast specialist in the Army probably had it better than the same job in civilian life. At any rate, you did not have to worry about being fired, laid off or boredom from lack of work. Fort Sill, Oklahoma had a large compliment of training. When you have training in the military, you also have injuries. There you have it, work. I worked in the cast room, pulled periodic call, and scrubbed in for surgery. Much time spent on casts for routine sprains of the ankle and clubfoot casts for neonates. I spent time studying because each year we had to take a military occupation specialty test. The test consisted of the following areas. See the example shown below. Evaluations were done yearly within our Military specialty. This was consonant with an evaluation filled out by your supervisor and signed off by the officer in charge or company commander, if I remember correctly. The one shown has a designation MOS[11] as 451.2, at that time considered non-medical. Later this designation was changed to a 91 series, which was medical.

MOS EVALUATION DATA REPORT (AR 611-203 · AR 138-305)		EVALUATION PERIOD AUG 64	USAEEC REFERENCE TCO SYMBOL 231	ROSTER NUMBER P 2883
SECTION 1. INDIVIDUAL EVALUATED.				
THRU: COMMANDING OFFICER 4A 4050 US ARMY HOSPITAL SILL FT OK		MOS IN WHICH EVALUATED 451.2		MOS EVALUATION SCORE 113
TO: RUSSELL WILLIAM		GRADE - PAY GRADE - PPD SP5 E-5	SERVICE NUMBER RA 56 344 735	
SECTION 2. INDIVIDUAL'S MOS EVALUATION TEST PROFILE.				

	SUBJECT MATTER AREA (DA PAM 12-451, DATED FEB 64)	VERY LOW	LOW	TYPI-CAL	HIGH	VERY HIGH
I	ANATOMY AND PHYSIOLOGY				X	
II	CARE AND HANDLING ORTHOPEDIC PATIENTS				X	
III	ORTHOPEDIC CONDITIONS			X		
IV	ORTHOPEDIC CAST ROOM MATERIALS, BANDAGES, MOLDS			X		
V	ORTHOPEDIC CAST ROOM TRACTION, FRAMES, BLUEPRINTS			X		
VI						
VII						
VIII						
IX						
X						

EPEECO FORM 10 1 MAY 64   SUPERCEDES AGTL-Q FORM 10 1 NOV 60 WHICH IS OBSOLETE   DISTRIBUTION: ORIGINAL - INDIVIDUAL'S 201 FILE FIRST COPY - INDIVIDUAL EVALUATED SECOND COPY - SPECIAL   FIRST COPY

My two years at Fort Sill, Oklahoma were relatively benign. I spent a great deal of time studying and working. At that time, we were working ½ day on Saturday. Therefore, I kept busy learning my trade. I grew to love orthopaedics, and today, still do. I was to take a big jump the first part of 1965; I was to be stationed in camp Zama, Japan.

This would be the first time I ever walked in a foreign land, though it would not be the last. Aside from the fact that I did not speak Japanese, everything else at Camp Zama Japan was

---

[11]   Military Occupational Specialty.

relatively easy to live with. It would be here that I began to develop a style in teaching, and making lesson plans, films, and devices to support my class. To give you an idea I submit below a copy of a document written for me by the doctor I worked with. This would be a beginning of my search for self. At the age of 32, I was just beginning to get a glimpse of what I was to become.

DEPARTMENT OF THE ARMY
HEADQUARTERS, UNITED STATES ARMY HOSPITAL, CAMP ZAMA, JAPAN
APO 96343

ZAH-Ortho   29 August 1967

SUBJECT: Recommendation for Advanced Medical Specialist School

TO: Commanding Officer
           Medical Company
           USAH Camp Zama, Japan
           APO 96343

1. It is recommended that Sp5 William J. Russell, RA56244735 be accepted to the Advanced Medical Specialist School.

2. Sp5 Russell has been under my supervision for twenty-two months during which time he has demonstrated the ability and desire to do any task well. He is consistently striving to find better or more efficient methods and as a result is one of the most knowledgeable orthopedic specialists I have known.

3. Sp5 Russell has been a medic for nine years working four years as a corpsman on general medical and neuropsychiatric wards and for five years as an orthopedic technician. Proficiency pay test scores are as follows:
                    Neuropsychiatric specialist ... 128
                    Medical specialist 116
                    Orthopedic specialist .... 113, 120 and 117

During his present assignment he has voluntarily given over 44 hours of instructions to the hospital staff, the majority of which were on orthopedic subjects. In conjunction with this, at his own expense, he has made three training movies and other aids to supplement the available material.

4. Sp5 Russell has demonstrated an active interest in patient care including a willingness to work many additional hours when required. He inhesitatingly makes suggestions to improve patient care which have often been helpful to the treating physician.

5. Sp5 Russell is a career soldier who potentially is capable of more than his current rank. He maintains himself physically and is emotionally stable. It is felt his potential to the service could be more fully realized following completion of this school.

ROBERT G. BUMP
Major, MC
Chief, Orthopedic Service

First, a little about Japan—I spent many long hours working as a cast specialist. Often there would be casualties from Viet

Nam, and there would be long hallways of litters with soldiers cast laden. It was our job, one other cast tech and myself, to make them ready for surgery. This would entail taking off their casts, or cutting the cast so that the doctor could view the wound. After surgery, the whole process repeated again, putting on a cast, or making a kind of open cast or splint to tend to the wound beneath. It was an arduous task, made more difficult by the fact that these were men, who had given much for their country, had often lost a limb.

I was tasked with the job of giving bandage and splinting classes as part of our yearly emergency first-aid requirement. All medical personnel were required to take classes every year as part of their training in emergency medical care. I traveled do different posts in Japan always giving the same class that I updated each year. I made 8mm movies to supplement my lecture material and some slides as well. In all, it was great fun and a learning experience that paved the way to my teaching style, knowledge, and self-knowledge, a search that would inevitably shape my destiny.

After those three years, I entered a specialized school. It was a 40 week advanced specialist course given at Beaumont General Hospital El Paso, Texas. This was an intense course. It gave us about two years of information crammed into 40 weeks. An advanced medical specialist is about as far as you can go in the army unless you become a nurse, a PA, or doctor. Unfortunately, all this training only equates to the level of a licensed vocational nurse in civilian life. Oh well, less means less responsibility. After these 40 weeks, I was ordered to Fort

Leonard Wood, Missouri. I started out in the education and training branch. Evidently, many of their advanced specialists were not doing well enough on the yearly required testing within their specialty. I was assigned to give refresher classes to all 91Cs (advanced clinical specialists). Again, I made training films. In fact, I was able to use some of the ones that I had made in Japan. This job was short lived however. I made the error of replying in some correspondence to another office with a signature block /for/ major so-and-so/—boy was she pissed. I thought that I was just doing my job. You know the old adage, show initiative and you are wrong. I was ordered to the night shift on the (URI) upper respiratory ward. After a few months of listening to young recruits hacking and coughing, I was assigned to the combination dental and orthopaedic ward.

Just prior to the orthopaedic/dental ward assignment there was an incident on the URI ward that needs mentioning. One morning, probably about two AM, I was passing medication on four wards of about 30 patients each. On my second ward, there were several recruits with high temperatures. I really did not have a lot of time to give each person special care. I corralled a patient that was on the mend to help me. I told him that he could walk with the patient with the high temperature to the shower and help him take a tepid shower, one of the ways to help reduce his fever along with the aspirin that I gave him. Thinking that this would be adequate, I made my way out to the long corridor to the next ward. As I was walking away, I noticed that I was hearing a little voice in my head warning me. Oh hell, I thought, I really need to get these meds passed. As I walked, further I heard running footsteps behind me.

Now the hair was standing up on the back of my neck. I turned around. It was the person that I had given the duty to walk the patient to the shower. He told me that I had better come back that there had been an accident. When we got back the patient was laying on the floor, blood all around his mouth, moaning in pain. Evidently, he had begun to faint, the person holding his arm tried to hold him up, and he swung him into a mental bed frame, mouth first. My dumb question was to ask why he did not tell me before. His answer was if he had been well, he would not have been there in the first place. Obviously, we had him sent to the emergency room and he ended up on the dental side of the ward I later worked. He had broken his jaw. In addition, I was the one who would be giving him his intramuscular antibiotics. Wouldn't you know it? I kept waiting for the court martial, the article 15, some kind of punishment, but no word, no punishment, no nothing. On the day that he was to be discharged from the ward, and the Army, he approached me. He said he thought at first I was a f—up, but after watching me for those many weeks, he was sure that I was an excellent medic. Besides, he had gotten his teeth fixed and gotten out of the army. Thanked me, smiled, and turned and left. It should be noted, the reason no charges were ever brought had to do with me having four wards to pass up 120 patient medications. Can you imagine what a defense lawyer would have done with that?

OK, what is learned here? First, we all have a gift for knowing when we should or should not do something. A nonschizophrenic voice will often warn us. For those who are not attuned to sound, but sight, perhaps a vision in their mind. Nevertheless, we are often given warnings prior to happenings.

The most difficult thing is being able to act upon those warnings. How many of you can wake yourself up when you are having a bad dream? All these abilities may lie dormant unless you do something about it.

Meaning Point

Communication with self at the unconscious level most often lies dormant. One of the basic paradigms in psychology has to do with the belief that certain communications from within our self are blocked. These communications brought to consciousness during stress, by an unknown stimulus or in the form of a flashback, by an unknown element(s) in the environment. This is especially true for the sense of smell.

CHAPTER FIVE

Communication and Living

The process of learning about self comes slow. There may be a set number of steps that one goes through that indicate a level of perception and maturation. I call these steps a theory of consequence in a hierarchy of learning.

HIERARCHY OF LEARNING
Theory of Consequence

7. **Change in behavior**
6. **Feedback**
5. **Need (motivation)**
4. **Psychological selectivity**
3. **Language**
2. **Awareness of others**
1. **Awareness of self**

Like Maslow's hierarchy of needs, each level builds upon itself. At the highest point, in my hierarchy, change in behavior should be the most up to date and ethically mature response to the situation at hand.

Awareness of Self

Obviously, this takes place at a very young age, and is therefore fraught with all the concomitants of Freudian theory. Lest we make more than we need of an already too complex subject, let us just admit that there is a lot we do not yet understand. On that note, let us begin with some of the things that we think do happen. We begin with the exploration of our body, our surroundings, and the people closest to us, our parents. It is not a quantum leap to interject that we make assessments based on these primary sense experiences. At some point, we recognize that we exist apart from others. This may be our first attempt to communicate our needs. What happens at this level may have a profound effect on the next step in the hierarchy.

Awareness of Others

The primary other should be our mother or mother figure for those of us adopted at an early age. It is postulated that we project from parental experience outward. In this way, we fashion what we see in others from the known persona of our primary parent figure. This process may cause us to treat others as we do our parents; be blind to the projection that we make upon another personality. It may be a safe process as long as our relationship with our parent is healthy. There is always a chance that we create a false identity. That we project upon another attributes that belong only to our parent, a process that may blind us to the actual personality of the person in question. This may be quite safe until the time when language takes on an importance in the personality asserting itself.

Language

With language comes a place to hang your thoughts, and store them in the complex circuitry of the brain. With smell, sound, and sight we can relive any happening of past life, with olfaction having the most power to create a past image or happening. When you talk to yourself, you use your language, the words that paint the picture of your world. Albeit, there are those that think in pictures, and others that use sound to remember, but for most of us we think with our language. Having said that, we still need to explain why this level is important. It is a matter of words. The number of words one has is like having money, the more you have, the more you have to spend; and therefore, the more of something you can acquire. That something is knowledge. If you have 2000 or 3000 words by the time you are 4 or 5 years old, you can better relate to others. Your vocabulary is your way into the world. The kind of words that you use often equates with your intelligence or capacity to understand others. This then, is your way into the social world. It is the first major step in being able to relate to others. By the time you reach 25, you have learned 95% of your vocabulary, that is, unless you do something about it. Imagine a child of 5 years who has already reached his 95%, but with an expansive vocabulary. Would he be a genius? Perhaps he would, but it would be impossible for most to relate to him because of the very nature of his gift. He would be beyond most in the thinking department. Therefore, language sets the stage for the next logical part of our hierarchy, namely psychological selectivity.

Psychological Selectivity

Why does anyone choose to do a particular thing? Why do some select nursing for a profession while others choose mechanics? You have bought your wife a fine jewel bracelet as a birthday gift, and the TV shows an ad about the very one that you have gotten, you feel as if she could guess just by looking at the commercial. You feel like she can read your mind. She cannot. However, the sweat rolling down your cheeks speaks differently. The concept of the lie detector relays a similar process. Your mind, keyed to respond to certain words that have value to only you. That selection process has psychological significance. It can be both a bother and a blessing.

What the process does normally is to keep us focused. It also allows us the ability to abstract from reality. We can put like things together and separate those things that do not belong in a group. It can cause us to focus on a life's work. It can be a part of our creative nature. Alternatively, it can become an obsession so compulsive that it destroys us. Which is it to be? It may have something to do with our need, our motivation.

Need, Motivation

You slept all night. What is the first thing that you do when you wake up? Right, a physiological need usually makes itself known, which causes a certain behavior. In most communication processes, we exchange information. Communication is not limited to just words, but many other factors as well.

It is necessary to separate need from motivation. For want of simplicity, a need for this writing shall imply returning the body to homeostasis[12]. A motivation, on the other hand, will imply psychological valence. Motivation comes from past learning about self. It is one's ability to choose a want. I am motivated to the degree that I know what I want to do in my life; and, to the degree that experience has pushed me.

Feedback

All communication requires a feedback loop to qualify as an interchange of information. Even those who talk to themselves require an answer to their spoken words, often spoken as if another was answering. These kinds of mutterings and other such non-schizophrenic voices in one's head assist in conversation sanity when there is no other to listen. The result is the same, a feedback loop is necessary.

The process is—message → sender → receiver → message decoded → reply (encoded). The feedback in this notation is the reply. Not all feedback is in the form of a verbal reply[13].

Definition of Communication

The ability of one person to change the behavior of another by using language, a body motion, an olfactory message, or in a

---

[12] Physiological and emotional equilibrium.
[13] A better model is given on page 15, *The Key to Survival*, by Smith, Tague-Busler, fourth edition, 2012.

way (written or verbal) that the forgoing process of message to sender is accomplished.

Change in Behavior

This is the acme of the hierarchy, the highest point of achievement in communication. Being fully achieved gives one the best chance of changing behavior in another. Changing behavior is what we do to survive. We change behavior of others on many levels, but written and verbal communication is the means for producing time gathering, the process that connects the past with the present. Connecting the past with the present should prevent us from repeating the same errors. It does not. This does not change the importance of this point once reached. An overall view of the communication process follows.

Many have written of the importance of semantic, pragmatic, and syntactic use within the communicative process. What also needs to be included is the importance of touch, olfaction, and the use of other senses to acquire meaning. Communication is not just the connection between two minds with words, but equally as well the connection of two bodies with chemical messages sent simultaneously as a result of the interaction between the two human polarities during the process of communication.

Humans have long since lost their claim to total bestiality; but some behaviors linger on as vestigial remains from a primal consciousness. These behaviors may push their way to the surface of our being in periodic flurries as behaviors designed to protect us from the insults of daily living, both in body and in word. These distance-reducing behaviors serve as an important device to ward off minor anxieties and place nametags on items being processed at the moment of occurrence.

A hierarchical arrangement of distant reducing behavioral spaces exists. [1] The stage of known distance by sight, or stage of eye contact called the sight space. [2] The stage of verbal contact, both written and spoken and, [3] the stage of touch and olfaction, called distance reduction zero. Each one of these stages, or spaces, is usually processed, or passed through, in the order mentioned. When processed in the forgoing fashion certain outcomes can be inherent. The primary outcome is the reduction of tension between the two polarities created by the act of communication. The reduction of anxiety, better understanding, and mental health are possible when the process is healthy, all favorable residuals of a positive communicative process.

Living Space—The Stage of Known Distance

Each creature upon this earth is in touch with an outside reality with its living space. A boundary defines the creature as a cell, a microbe, or a person. Within specific boundaries of each human, there exist separate spaces that allow each one to process the oncoming events of living. Crowding these spaces may cause one to have a fight on one's hands. Ignore these spaces and be thought of as insensitive, or worse. For some these spaces are vast, and for others these spaces are small. In our western culture, 18 inches is the point of comfort or that distance one might be able to tolerate another's presence. This does not include how one processes the distance reduction up to that point. At some point in each of our spaces, we take notice of everything alive or in motion. This aspect of something *being noticed* should command our attention. For whatever reason when we take notice of something on the fringe of our living space, we have begun the primary stages of communication and distance reduction zero. We can call this process psychological selectivity, preconditioning, or stimulus response activation, but the significant feature is that it is a stage of communication for man and many animals. The observations that we make during the preliminary stages of approach behavior are a special kind of nonverbal communication. These actions, gestures, facial expressions, and other bodily behaviors give clue to our present emotional state and either open or close channels to further distance reduction.

There are several spaces surrounding each of use. We have a sight space, a voice space, and a contact space. The sight space is the largest. When one enters our sight space, we may take perfunctory notice, or if this person is known to us, we have the option of looking, ignoring, or using some gesture to decrease the distance between us. If one heeds our signal, one may then move into our second space, our voice space. One may then listen to the sound of our voice, see our facial expression, or expression of posture, and if all seems well, venture into our last space, the space of possible contact and the space of insensible perspiration loss, a space that allows one to decipher pheromones. Moreover, all this time during the process, it has been towards *distance reduction zero*. Any movement in the opposite direction would have a negative effect on total communication insofar as it would increase distance rather than decrease distance between the two personality poles.

The process of moving through the spaces is the part of the initial communicative response, without it, communication ceases to exist. A problem is that some may view the process of speaking as communication, leaving out the intrinsic relationship that exists within the circumscribed living spaces, especially the one of contact with concomitant exposure to another's chemical messages. To communicate well means to be able to adjust to the demands of each space in an order that is different for each person contacted, while maintaining some consistency within the verbal medium. What this means is that we will have to use language as our base in sending messages, usually as words. However, it also means that we should be aware that some of our emotional responses are colored beyond our conscious control, where words are a very bloodless substitute for the feelings deep within our conscious being, ones hidden from view by our conscious awareness.

Developing Meaningful Dialogues

To reduce the tension, the anxiety of living as a separate entity, to become closer to the condition experienced as feeling good about self, I have mentioned that we need to develop meaningful dialogues with significant others. This concept entails within its confines as a philosophic approach the need for language as a tool for understanding. In man, this language is the most prominent feature of being human. For to be human is to speak, but to be most human of all is to communicate about the past, the future, and doing this while existing in the present. Then, acquiring a developmental dialogue within the world of people in the world of things is also a process of placing self in a working relationship environment that is dynamic, always changing, a flow of events and people in the fluid of time. Further, these relationships must be with significant others, people whom we trust, respect, yes even love. Finally, we will have to understand something about how we communicate in the world of words, both spoken and written, and in the way that nonverbal signals emanate from the body.

Word Ownership

Who owns the words that we speak? Certainly we should be held accountable for the symbols we utter; yet, many of us each day are willing to use words, special jargon, and word orientations beyond our own comprehension (like a parrot), without feeling that any crime against understanding has been committed. Word ownership implies certain responsibilities of the user. Each user needs to be aware of the possible consequences of the verbal or written symbols in a particular environment, context, syntax, or orientation, their relationship to each other regarding the experience of the listener's education, native tongue, culture, and any variation of mental state of the listener while having full awareness of the need to formulate and evaluate feedback.

Our responsibility goes beyond the mere speaking of words; it denotes to each language user the importance of the need to be aware of word orientation on many levels of abstraction.[14] Word ownership suggests that we must take credit for each word we use, while taking into consideration that we were not the primary formulator of the word as in "words are the coins of the realm," we use what others have created before us. We are only the spender and an intermediate receptacle shaping the word to our needs of the moment. What awareness should create in us is the understanding that we can be held accountable for the words we speak if we do four things. First, know what the word means. Second, create a living context to support the word. Third, use correct enunciation so that the listener can identify the word. Fourth, utilize feedback to clarify or add meaning to the word when necessary.

The Notion of Meaning

The notion of meaning first resides within the self and next in the formation of the word. In order to understand a meaning we must place our self into contact with words. Agreement between users is acquired by the usage of a common tongue containing units of meaning put together to form a thought, denotation/connotation, or identify a past agreement in a previous learned language or system of symbols. However, the meaning will ultimately reside within the self-first, then be projected outside of the person for confirmation and placement against the language in use.

---

[14] *People in Quandaries,* Johnson, Wendell, Harpers & Brothers, NY & London, 1946, pg 99.

Word or symbol (sign) usage is a process that frees us from the drudgery of manipulating cumbersome objects/concepts, but instead allows us to let something quite small and intangible in the macroscopic sense represent something outside in the physical world of things and people. The essential danger with any such symbol or sign usage is in the user's possible loss of objectivity insofar as the user may identify the word with the thing, or the user may act as if the word was the thing itself. In addition to this problem, and sometimes more serious, is the user's unawareness of the level of abstraction, using high level meanings to make reference to low level functions as in using the word love to represent the contact communication of coitus.

An example of the aforementioned identification with the word as the thing it symbolizes demonstrated by doing the following experiment. Take several 5 x 7 index cards and print the following words on them so that the size of each letter is two inches high: God, dirt, Jesus, Mother, earth, dog, wife, feces, and the word this. Place these cards word side up on the floor in no special array. Pick someone at random to come to you and follow these instructions. Go to the cards and pick one out without picking the card up. Take you foot and stamp on the card as if to grind it into the ground with your heel. After you have done this, bring the card to a place and dispose of it; as for instance a wastebasket. You can either have the same person continue to do this until he/she refuses or pick a different person for each card. Keep track of the order that the cards the brought back to you. Have the person hold the card up for all to see. You will notice that most of the time you will have a pattern (diagram 1).

Diagram 1

1.	A.	dirt	2.	A.	this	3.	A.	earth
	B.	this		B.	dirt		B.	dirt
	C.	earth		C.	earth		C.	this

4.	A.	feces	5.	A.	Mother	6.	A.	Jesus
	B.	dog		B.	wife		B.	feces

7.	A.	God

Notice that the first three A groups are words that can be stepped on without "hurting" them so to speak. B groups almost the same. C groups, last resort, or a person who does not care. When you identify the word as the thing, it follows that you must treat the symbol as the thing. The numbers represent the choices of cards as they are brought back with the letters representing variations of the first three choices.

If one understands that another may become quite defensive when his choice of words are challenged, or that one may react to an abstraction that we are unaware, then it would seem a better approach if one seeks the direction of understanding by forming agreements and merging contexts. Without agreement between language users meaning becomes an obscure form without shape or substance, an entity forever elusive and hidden from view, a gray mouse that scurries in the night sought by many, caught by few.

Touch, Towards Distance Reduction Zero

Behavior that reduces distance between polarities is healthy and behavior that increases distance is potentially harmful by increasing stress. This is better understood when one regards distancing between polarities due to anger. The human organism has an inherent polarity for all humankind, it might be called the capacity to love, so that any behavior that does not satisfy this basic need to love and comfort through touch could be thought of as maladaptive or potentially harmful by causing aloneness. Aloneness is a product of the mind insofar as the perception of self is an important aspect in the process of the determination of what constitutes an alone state.

The concept of self is identified, expanded, and abstracted from the exogenous reality by using language. Listening to the nonschizophrenic voices within our mind or talking to self can be a process of identifying an aloneness state of being. What we know about our self is a proprioceptive[15] truth firsthand, then projected outwardly to those about us with words. Since no one can get into our mind and see the world through our eyes with our psychological modifications and neurochemical environment, all anyone knows about our personal self is what we wish to reveal.

A dichotomy exists within our personal self. Self is experienced in a functional and organic way. Awareness of self in the functional sense implies emotional and cognitive activity.

---

[15] The unconscious perception of movement and spatial orientation arising from stimuli within the body itself.

We are aware that we exist alone because we think alone, there are no outside thoughts clouding our inner world aside from the ones we cause (schizophrenia excluded). When thoughts come to us from the outside world, they are usually in some form of communication. These communications will symbolize something in the world of people and the world of events. Our awareness, our ability to communicate with others, will have a relationship to our mental self as well as will the meanings invested in the words that are used. We must be able to identify ourselves as a separate entity from the world of concepts built of words. When we place our mental hand against the wall of conceptual things, we must be able to feel where the wall begins and ourselves end or else move in a world of uncertainties clouded by imperfect boundaries; a symptom of schizophrenia.

Awareness of self in the organic sense comes to us as we have physical contact with the world of people and things. To touch is to have a very special kind of knowledge. Children learn this at a very early age. They explore the world of people and things with different parts of their body evoking pleasure and sometime pain, always learning something of the fundamental aspects of contact communication. All reduction of space between individuals can ultimately lead to contact in the physical sense. This contact is the final step in nonverbal communication. Contact often reveals what words fail to say.

It is said that sexual contact to orgasm brings us as close and as far away as we may ever be. The result of sexual contact is perhaps the ultimate in a feedback loop, each sensation creating a response in the sharing organism and a process that lessens physiological tension. For some coitus becomes the excuse for touch, better to have this brief touch than no touch at all. Sexual touch is a special form of communication that reaches into the very essence of being, our germ cell seeking to touch another's. We may have little or no control over this deep-seated process within. In the nature of a chemical equation we must fulfill our obedience to the call of primal fusion, that behavior being seen on the surface many times only the ripple caused by this fundamental force deep within our being, perhaps only a microscopic speck dictating to the total organism. Coitus may be an extreme example leaving out the myriad of possible contacts between organisms, but it may be the apriori of existence, that which first served our uniting to form another. The holding of one in love, the shake of a hand in friendship, the embrace between two friends, these are all examples of distant reducing behaviors.

Touch in the form of lying on of hands is a form of healing. Touch in this form is more than physical intimacy; it is the transmission of energy from one to another. In the form of massage, this deep touch causes the body to release endogenous endorphins, substances that act against pain and is the body's natural way of dealing with pain without the help of drugs.

The process of Kirlian[16] photography demonstrates that many individuals project flares of different colors from the distal most aspect of their fingers during emotional states. This appears to be physical evidence that the body does emit an

---

[16]   *Roots of Consciousness,* Mishlove, Jeffrey, Random House, NY, page 226.

energy force. What this force can do or how it fits in within the confines of communication is unknown at this time.

Olfaction, or When Molecules Mingle

A kind of olfactory knowledge exists when the contact space is entered, in that; it is possible for one to process the expired microscopic droplets of another's system. Obviously, olfaction in the sense that one can recognize something of the immediate surroundings is common to all, but more importantly, an intimate relationship may exist with the process within the body chemistry. This may be so even without the person being aware of this relationship or even understanding one's feelings when such close contact exists. As primitive beings we relied on our olfactory ability to relieve our sexual tensions and today there can still be seen a strong vestigial response during courting behaviors. Each person is in touch with his surroundings with a special chemical space that is the byproducts of that person's metabolic state. It is the body's internal biorhythm sending signals resulting from the present state of feeling, health, or process of disease. If this is so, then a kind of chemical relationship exists within one's own bloodstream communicated to another by way of expired air from the sending system and is a situation that creates a kind of exocrine effect. This form of primal communication is not self evident for it is a process that we have long since forgotten how to recognize.

An odor or smell or a scent consists of molecules of a volatile substance carried in the air, or for some aquatic animals carried in the water. The sense of smell is therefore the detection of chemicals. In the language of smell, odors are secreted by one animal and carried in the air or water to the olfactory organs of another animal of the same species. The odors act as messengers telling an animal about its fellows as in the examples of wild dogs, catfish and deer mice. These messengers called pheromones are analogous to hormones, the chemical messengers secreted by an internal gland and carried by the blood to affect distant parts of the body. The standard definition of a pheromone is that it is a substance, which is secreted to the outside of the body and received by a second individual of the same species in which it releases a specific reaction, for example, a definite behavior or developmental process.

Pheromones secreted in the urine, as in wild dogs, in the feces, as in the hippopotamus, which scatters its dung with its tail, from the mouth, as in food sharing by ants and bees; or pheromones secreted from special glands. Deer have pheromone secreting glands on their faces and hoofs and the queen bee secretes 'queen substance' from her mandibular glands. There are two kinds of pheromones. *Releaser* pheromones cause overt changes in an animal's behavior. If a minnow is injured it releases a pheromone that sends other minnows fleeing from the scene. The formic acid discharged by wood ants when their nest is disturbed brings other wood ants to their aid. *Primer* pheromones have general affect, altering the physiological state of other animals rather than changing their immediate behavior. Isolated female mice come into breeding condition when urine from male mice containing a primer pheromone was sprayed into their cages and 'queen substance' prevents the development of rival queens in the beehive by suppressing their development.

Researchers have been successfully trained to tell a person's sex by simply smelling their urine. On occasion, I can tell if a woman is pregnant just by smelling the urine before applying the HCG (pregnancy) test. Researchers have concluded that we have the capability to distinguish the subtleties between male and female pheromone but cannot do it automatically. Still, it must be that these chemical messengers have an effect upon every one of us. We just need to learn how to decipher them.

During the time of stress or when placed in a situation causing fear, one is made ready for fight or flight by a substance known as epinephrine secreted directly into our blood stream. This hormone stimulates the heart, constricts vessels, and in general, gets the body ready for some kind of action. Is it possible that the byproducts of this process can also be picked up by another system? If so, this may explain why one feels uneasy around one in stress or how one picks up the message of fear in the air.

The importance of the forgoing is within the idea that olfactory messages may be responsible for some of the maladaptive behavior that we see. When one is feeling strange, perhaps one should look to the surroundings for evidence of psychic turmoil in others, especially those in close quarters. When we feel empathy, how close will we be? Why can the simple closeness of another calm those experiencing unrest and anxiety? Distant reduction zero, touch, communication that calms, goes to a deeper level of our being.

More research is necessary on human behavior regarding the sense of smell and taste and their relation to emotion and feelings. Perhaps one focus for study is in the area of learning to identify behavior on a chemical level. If we can learn to identify internal states of others by merely decoding their chemical messages, we may be much closer to a fundamental form of communication. Chemical pictures may be worth ten thousand verbal words.

Some Working Principles

Pick up your dictionary, a pad and pencil and wander out into the world about you as if you were in a foreign land. Use caution when listening to people speak their minds. Trespass on the many spaces as if they were alive and pay heed to the unspoken as well as the spoken word. Become aware of the many meanings of words per se, for this awareness will keep you healthy and from making hasty judgments. Approach one in a way the he may give you signals allowing for space reduction. This will bring you through the three spaces in comfort creating a pleasurable contact with maximum tension reduction.

Each person in your immediate environment has potential for giving you tension relief. Your polarity will be determined as you approach. Should this process produce encroachment upon another or feelings of uneasiness within yourself stop your approach and evaluate the situation. You might stop within the voice space and listen for a warning growl. Sometimes it has only been your speed of entry; trying to take up the distance too quickly.

You should experiment with the process of distant reduction with known personalities. Having some knowledge of their personality will help you with future evaluations when making contact with unknown personalities. Learn to read the *yes, yes* in her eyes and pheromones when her lips are saying *no, no.* Become familiar with those who light up when they see you. Be able to identify positive signals in distance reduction from those who send these signals to you most often.

Remember the three spaces: sight, voice, and contact. One must see you first, then one should hear the sound of your voice, and then contact may, or may not, be allowed. If allowed, try to focus on the chemical messages during the closeness by clearing your mind of all thoughts. Inhale the scent of the person and wait for 16-18 seconds for a new feeling within yourself. It will take much practice to learn how to evaluate your feelings after entering the contact space.

A meaningful dialogue may be the result of a pleasurable contact after verbal communication has taken place. Moreover, it may be *this* touch that feeds our soul, the act of human contact in a world of space, and the temporary joining of separate nervous systems, sharing a powerful nonverbal experience in the viscosity of time.

CHAPTER SIX

THE HERE AND NOW OF BEING

There are those who enjoy life after the fact. I remember when I was young that my Mother would often say, "I know something you don't know." This usually meant that something good was going to happen in the near future. The problem was that she would not tell me. So, I would wonder what it was, and depending on the time of the year, would wait patiently until whatever it was would occur. Sometimes it was really nice and other times it was neutral, at least to me. It occurs to me that this may have something to do with my inability to, on occasion, enjoy the here-and-now.

How many times in your life have you had the thought that something you had experienced awhile back was great? However, during the time that the experience was happening, you really did not feel it; a kind of emotional anesthesia seemed to cloud the event. You moved through the event in a way that it did not register on your senses. This is what I call not being there. Emotional distancing may be a kind of defense mechanism created out of personal necessity. If you look back on your life, you may be able to remember a happening, a situation, or an event that caused you emotional pain. Perhaps your unconscious decided that this would never happen again and so created a shield, one that now interferes with situations having the same emotional tone. Moreover, what is worse, this emotional cold front can move into other areas of experience causing a distancing from the event, creating a not being there effect. This concept impinges on personality theory, and therefore, it would be best to review possible constructs that could explain the existence of a time delayed feeling toward experience.

The thought comes to mind, just what model would be best? A plethora of personality theories exist. Do any of the present-day theories explain how emotional distancing from the here and now comes into being? If so, which ones. One should have a basic assumption about the world in which he lives. An attempt to understand the world we live in is by nature, a human ability bound to the gift of psychesthesia[17]. We have an awareness of self. No theory is more profound to the understanding of this than the theory of psychoanalysis.

Under the heading of defense mechanisms, the psyche employs a variety of ways to defend. The ultimate aim of all defenses is to achieve repression. Freud stated two: primal repression and repression proper. Primal repression is the more archaic of the two. Freud suggested that there are elements within the id that can never reach consciousness. Therefore primal repression is little more that a historical reference. However, repression proper seems to be best understood as a process that pushes something into the unconscious to protect the ego or the present self. This process could also be responsible for the desensitizing of one from the now. It is as if your captain of the mind states, "shields up." While in

_____

[17] This word does not exist, per se; but a good translation would be an Awareness of self, as in sensation.

the protective state, communication may be in stasis and you cannot beam down to any other world, you are shielded for your protection. Aside from the star trek metaphor, what can you do to alleviate the situation?

The following table gives clue to the operation of the senses and the possibility that there is more to our senses than we often believe.

SENSE DATA RELATED TO STATES OF CONSCIOUSNESS

Senses	Conscious	Subconscious or Preconscious	Unconscious
Sight	What is seen, the Actual reality as In looking at a picture Or landscape, however Much is left out due to Psychological selectivity.	That not seen by the The unaided eye, as In body aura, or Beyond the normal Color range.	Latent image, after Image as in photo- Graphic memory For some the ability To see an image of Things no longer in The present.
Hearing	The actual sound, as in voice, bell, or wind.	Beyond the range of Hearing as in dog whistle.	Sound of fear, sound Emanating from an Object that no one Else can hear, often A warning.
Smell	The actual smell, as in A banana, perfume, Food cooking, or for Some the ability to Process pheromone.	Memory recall, as in Bring one back in time. Some may be able to Decode the droplet Particles from another Body.	Setting off the flight Or fight response Producing a panic Attack, pheromone Response.

Taste	The actual taste, as in Food, banana, orange, Licorice or coffee.	When crossing over to Smell may bring back Old memories, but May be limited to Short term memory.	**When crossing over To smell, may bring About similar Experience, but may Relate to long term Memory.**
Touch	The actual texture of an Object, thing or person, As well as temperature.	Latent qualities related To the objects Whereabouts, as in Being able to tell who Touched the object Last.	**Being able to pick up Qualities beyond the Here-and-now a Special knowledge About the person Who owned the Object as in persona, Good or bad karma.**

We are bound to our world by our senses. As fleeting as they may be, sensual stimuli constantly bombard us. It is indeed how we perceive our world. The sound of it, the color of it, the smell and taste of, and the feel of it; all together the world as we know it. No one else can see the world through our senses. It is but ours alone. If 20 people experience a happening, you have 20 different versions of that happening. Only trained observers are able to come together on agreement in terms of what they have seen, smelled, tasted, heard, or touched. However, there is a modicum of truth in any shared experience that one may infer. This then, is the basis for the stabilization of the here-and-now.

To be in the here-and-now one needs to focus on a sensation such as color, sound, or a sense with the strongest attraction for the event. If the event has to do with sound, focus on the quality, pitch, or nature of the sound. If the event has to do with sight, really see it. Study with intent to remember. In order for one to be there, it is important to gather the event with as many of the senses as is possible. This will mean that one has to focus with intent. I have found that talking to one's self often assists with remembering. However, to create the moment in the present time one must focus with the full array of senses.

To lock a situation with sensual impressions is to give it life in the now and to record the event for all time. Association with olfaction is the oldest for recall. For some music brings the past to life. Using all the senses at one time will make the event live in the memory of now.

Passive imprints happen during stress. If a situation happens that provokes a strong emotional response, one may carry the baggage of that feeling around for many years. Posttraumatic stress disorder is probably a byproduct of such events. Passive imprints are not acquired by intent to remember, they are attached to strong stimuli that have driven a heavy nail into the brain. You cannot help but remember. Flashbacks happen when a present environment contains many of the sensual elements of the original event. At once, you are there again. Often these flashbacks are accompanied by panic attacks as well. Therefore, the question is, "does being in the here-and-now present one with any adverse emotional flashbacks?"

A primary symptom in PTSD has to do with flashback phenomenology. So, I repeat the question, "does this type of here-and-now from the past present with an adverse effect?" Obviously, the answer should be yes. However, is it? I have sat in many groups. Sessions designed to assist one with recovery from emotional stress created by combat situations. Though limited to combat, the outcome is much the same as it would be from situations created from other than combat. Catharsis related to the process of therapeutic verbal ventilation may work for some, but not for me. After listening for hours as each in the group revisited the past, I became aware that nothing was changing. Pathology was only making new inroads within each persona. It was a mess. I see now how the psychiatrists of old made their money. Reliving the past does not necessarily assist with the present. In order to change ones internal being, one must use a cognitive approach; anything else is sub clinical. Of course, that is my opinion. Nevertheless, let us scrutinize this more closely.

What counts is the cognitive process, how one interprets his reality. One's belief system can be reinforced, alas, re-infected by thoughts produced in the present. As in the forgoing group therapy, situations relived ad infinitum. Albert Ellis, the founder of Rational-Emotive Therapy, was well aware of this fact. What I am suggesting is a deeper look into the possible cause. With a cognitive approach, one can become aware of faulty thinking. One can learn to control how he or she reacts to old messages, even ones that come into existence from past stimuli made active in the here-and-now. It is in the process of remembering that allows for change. While it is true that past memories can bring maladaptive behavior, it is also true that we do not have to allow old memories to hurt us anymore. With a cognitive approach, we can relearn and reload these memories in the light of the present. For example, your parents should not forever be the cause, or the excuse, for your present behavior. You can become responsible. However, this becomes more difficult when a stimulus/response situation occurs. What we call flashbacks in PTSD occur without conscious control. Can we change these behaviors with a so-called cognitive approach?

The dichotomy between controlled remembering and flashbacks while *being there* create an almost impossible concept to grasp. On the one hand, one needs not to be numb to certain past-experiences when they recur, yet still be able to disallow certain flashback experiences to surface causing a re-experience of an unpleasant happening. It is probably not possible to stop a flashback, but only modify how you react to it. The first time a flashback occurs, it is usually without warning. A kind of sense datum proclivity may exist between past and present experience with preponderance for one or more senses. This means that given a similar sensation experience as one that happened in the past can create a feeling like the one that happened in the past. If this is so, perhaps one can predict what experiential stimuli *might* produce a flashback. The next step would be to produce a safe environment for this feeling to be reborn.

I remember an example. I was working in a clinic as a nurse. On this particular warm summer day, a young Hispanic girl came to the clinic with an injury to her right forearm. She was crying. I kneeled down in front of her to examine her injury. With her dark brown eyes, tan skin, long black hair, she looked like a Vietnamese orphan that I once treated in Vietnam. As I looked into her tear-strewn face, with a warm breeze coming through the open window, the smell of fresh cut grass and perspiration down my back, the past jumped into the present. The sense datum lock had brought me back 27 years. At once, I was again in Vietnam looking into the face of an orphan created by war. It took several minutes to shake the realness of an experience that happened so long ago, as it was as real now as it had been then. I managed to bring myself to the present and finish what I had started, but the feeling stayed with me the rest of the day.

In the environment of the clinic, one might say I was safe. I was safe because there was strong anchorage to the present. My job, the physical setting, the people (aside from the girl), all presented my senses with stimuli contrary to the flashback. In a word, I was *rooted* in the present with only a wisp of the past flooding my senses. The key to safeness has to do with awareness. To the degree that one is aware, one is able to contain the feelings brought about by a flashback. However, often there is a concomitant panic attack. When this happens, there is a feeling of some vague threat or a sense of stark terror. Flashbacks and panic attacks are related, but not always discernible as being concomitant. It goes back to the theory of psychoanalysis with emphasis on repression proper. As a defense mechanism, repression holds back certain memories that might be painful or contrary to the belief system. However, perhaps after a time the hold on the memory may become weak, thus allowing another occurrence to drag it to the surface of consciousness.

A spontaneous thought erupts into consciousness. Perhaps a word comes to mind, one for which you have lost the meaning. In the process of remembering the meaning, any thought associations are filed with less data. This may be an example of the brain defragging. The process of free association may be such a process, when guided by an outside individual; perhaps, psychoanalysis was just a way of doing this, maybe Freud was further ahead of his time than he ever knew. The only danger in this process may be in therapy groups where individuals continue to spew the same sewage repeatedly, without discarding damaging content.

The next chapter shall delve into the three parts of the personality. I do not know how many pay attention, but our world often comes in threes. From the concept of Id, Ego, and Superego to the Father, the Son and the Holy Ghost, the trichotomies of life abound.

CHAPTER SEVEN

THREE PILLARS OF LIFE

Spirit	Organic	Knowledge
Religion	*Body*	*Mind*
God	*Flesh*	*Psyche*
Soul	*Chemical*	*Logos*
Weightless	*Carbon*	*Reason*
Eternal	*Finite*	*Tentative*
psychospiritual	**psychochemical**	**psychointellectual**

The foregoing relates to the three parts of the personal self: psychospiritual, psychochemical, and psychointellectual orientations to organic reality, a kind of alpha-omega sequence in life. The three pillars denote aspects of what are *spirit, organicity,* and *knowledge.* While each state exists as part of the whole, each is acted upon by the mind as a central core to being, ideally balanced by having equal representation for each third of the total personality. However, in real life this is seldom the case. Often one aspect will dominate. This can be seen especially so in situations of love relationships. Ascension to a higher plane of existence will be within one or more of the pillars, and to the extent, that one dominates, shown as a persistence of personality trait, or the individual psychological selectivity;

not always at the conscious level. This is often what separates mediocrity from greatness.

A Higher Plane

In the process of ascension through life, one should reach the highest level of achievement that one can in each of the three pillars of life. I have chosen a few concepts in each pillar to serve as anchors, words that identify qualities that relate to that part of the triad. Starting with the psychochemical pillar, these thoughts come to mind.

Psychochemical Orientation to Organic Reality

Starting from zygote, we ascend to adulthood. In the process of becoming, one should tend toward perfection. Our DNA code is given. We are only now finding ways to decode DNA and predict organic reality as it pertains to human form and being. Within the limits, that now exist, we should make every attempt to be the best that we can. From the point of view of *body, flesh, carbon* this has to do with diet, exercise, medicine, and periodic medical examinations. What you do to your physical body will determine your life ascension. Life is *finite*; however, these boundaries are extended every decade. We can live longer in better health if we choose to do so. Our body is a *chemical* environment. Knowing something about that environment may keep one healthy; therefore, learn.

Psychointellectual Orientation to Organic Reality

Mind over matter, thought provoked well being. Sounds a little futuristic, but it is not. We have known for decades that psychological well being equates with good health. The illegitimate child of philosophy, psychology, came into being out of the need to explain human nature, to quantify that which is unquantifiable, to predict ones emotional states. Today a plethora of books containing many theories exists; our present day tower of babble. From an eclectic point of view, select what works for you. Each of us has a vision of how we think the world is. Having an awareness of that internal view and the way it fits with the true reality of existence gives the best quest for truth. How one lives, one's life is as important as what one believes, for the two are often inseparable. Therefore, one should continue their education at all costs. Knowledge is *tentative* at best, for all things change. Stagnation of the brain chemistry leads to recursion. That which is not used goes into terminal atrophy.

Psychospiritual (also psychespiritual) Orientation to Organic Reality

One cannot escape the wonder of the world. Whether pragmatist, egotist, agnostic, atheist, or God fearing, we all walk this earth. It rains on believers and unbelievers alike. One once said that if you lived your life like there was no God, you had better hope that you are right. This is not a place to preach, but a place to point out that you have a choice. Some believe in order to spiral upward in this pillar that a belief system is necessary, be it God, a supreme force, or an eternal logos. People who have ascended to the acme of this pillar have strived to better humankind, namely: Martin Luther King Jr., Red Skeleton, Anwar Sadat, Mother Teresa, Albert Einstein, and many others. It would seem that few attain the highest stage of moral development.[18] Some would argue that there is no unconditional moral law that applies to all rational beings, one that is independent of any personal motive or desire. They would argue that everyone has a motive, a desire, or psychological bent in a certain direction. However, isn't that what comprises the substance of the three pillars? In some way, the personal self is a reflection of dominance whether in one pillar, or all three divided in some way. What you see mirrored in the personality is strongly tinted by the psychospiritual, psychochemical, or the psychointellectual. We need an example to make this better understood.

Since we are within the psychospiritual frame of reference, an example that defines that domain would be best.

The Case of John

John Doe was a God-fearing man, often times to the extreme. He believed profusely in the golden rule, do unto to others as you would have them do unto you, but do it first. He proclaimed of the Lord Almighty aloud in the midst of others often, and he went to church almost every Sunday. However, he had issue with the fact that not everyone believed as he did. He would spend time in conversation trying to convince others, especially his close friends. This would often lead to long periods

---

[18]   Lawrence Kohlberg (1971)

when he would not hear from anyone, not even his close friends. Eventually, he became somewhat of a recluse. One Sunday while attending church service, he noted that the sermon did not agree with some of his underlying principles. He stood abruptly and gave argument, openly and loudly. This eventuated in John leaving the church in a huff. He was no longer welcome in the congregation. More a recluse than ever, he developed agoraphobia and finally was deeply in need of professional help.

The case of John is to the extreme. As is the case with many personality disorders John's focus is an exaggeration of the normal. We all have underlying issues with reality, people, organizations, but with restraint. We have a modicum of control. We obey societal rules for the most part. The psychospiritual part of the personal self should intermingle within the triad, thereby creating conscience, perhaps even a moral being. To the degree that one part of the personal self is dominate, to that degree is reflected the kind of person seen on the surface and in touch with life.

We each should be in touch with our personal self. Being strong in belief but weak in knowledge may cause failure in achieving our goal in life; and if we neglect our body, a life cut short, may be the result.

CHAPTER EIGHT

ARRIVAL

I often think of that person who worked all his life to achieve fame and wealth. Having done so by the age of 50 he looked down upon the many below him, he had nowhere to go, not only that, he was not now certain that he liked where he was.

I truly believe that men do not begin to mature until about 60. Well, hopefully a little before that. It all depends on what you mean by mature. In terms of the three pillars of life, it would mean that in each area of the personal self that one has achieved the most that he or she could, given the basic ingredients necessary to do so.

Arrival for me has been the result of many factors, not the least of which is the military. A good reason for including my resume, has to do with my belief that one should show a reason why anyone should take anything they say to heart.

Background:

January 1959 to December 1962:

Neuropsychiatric specialist Letterman Army Medical Center, San Francisco, California. Working as a psych-tech on a neurosurgery ward and closed psychiatric ward. I did direct patient care to include tracheotomy care, skin care of the paraplegic and multiple sclerosis patients and head trauma patients. Complete bed care and assistance with all bed frames.

January 1963 to September 1968:

I worked as an orthopaedic specialist: two years clinical Fort Sill, Oklahoma and three years surgical orthopaedics while stationed in Japan. Primary duties: cast care, traction set up, skin care, pulmonary toilet and personal hygiene. Additionally, taught emergency fracture care to nonmedical personnel using a film that I made.

February 1968 to September 1969:

Department of nursing as education administrator and coordinator, Fort Leonard wood Army Hospital. Additionally, working on an upper respiratory infection ward and an orthopaedic ward passing medication and as treatment nurse.

September 1969 to September 1970:

Vietnam as combat medic working in a clearing station (like MASH); acting battalion surgeon for one month.

September 1970 to September 1974:

Acting as drug and alcohol counselor 47th combat support hospital (MASH), Fort Lewis, Washington. Additionally, working on orthopaedic ward with amputee patients passing medication and doing treatments as required.

September 1974 to June 1980:

Teaching at the Patient Care Specialist Course Madigan Army Medical Center Tacoma, Washington. Disciplines taught include medical terminology, psychology, orthopaedic diseases and casting techniques to include methods of traction for fracture care. Supervising students in the clinical areas of: orthopaedic ward, surgical clinic, dermatology clinic, students passing medications, and doing all minor procedures assigned. This includes working in a medical clinic screening a military sick call. Last six months of 1980 and the first five months of 1981, I worked at Western State Hospital, Tacoma, Washington, on a closed psychiatric ward. Duties included working with the chronically mentally ill, passing medication and doing required treatments.

June 1981 to November 1986:

Comprehensive Mental Health Center, Tacoma, Washington 98403. I worked as a nurse/counselor. I had a caseload of 30 clients. My primary duty was as a case manager for the Community Support Team.[19] My primary duties, for the client's, included supervision of all care, home visits, medication administration, to include Prolixin, and acting as an advocate for clients living in the community.

---

[19] The Community Support Team Concept can be found on line as CST, Team Based Services. I have been trying to get one started in Mendocino County, California as a mental health board member since 2013.

Evening work September 1983 to November 1986:

Teaching at Knapp Business College, Tacoma, Washington 98403. Taught the following disciplines: Medical terminology, psychology related to motivation, insurance and coding, business communications, and an introduction to supervision.

November 1986 to July 1992:

Mental health Clinical Services Associate as Quality Assurance/Utilization Review Coordinator for Mendocino County Mental Health Services, Ukiah, California. Additionally, I worked in the day treatment (adult) program as an LVN & psych-tech doing various groups.

July 1992 to February 1993:

Working as Director of Staff Development for Care West Manzanita (long term care facility) Cloverdale, California 95425. Duties included orientation of new employees, in-service program and pre-certification program for CNA's; instruction for NA's to become CNA's (Certified Nursing Assistants).

February 1993 to March 1996:

I returned to Mendocino County Mental Health as utilization review coordinator.

October 1987 to May 2008:

Teaching medical terminology class at Mendocino Community College, Ukiah, California. Have self published a book with the title, "Medical Terminology by the Mnemonic Story System." The book can be purchased from Xlibris Corporation, or Amazon.com.

October 1998 to February 2006:

I worked as an LVN Potter Valley Community Health Center, part time.

Education:

Willits High School
Willits, California
Graduated June 1952

Fort Steilacoom Community
College
Tacoma, Washington
Associate Arts and Science
Graduated October 1978

Saint Martin's College
Lacey, Washington 98503
BA Psychology
Graduated May 1982

Bryson University
Columbus, Mississippi
Master of Arts in Education
June 8, 2010

---

[20] The Bryson University degree-granting program is in conformity with the requirements of the National Distance Learning Accreditation.

Military Education:

Neuropsychiatric Specialist Course
Letterman Army Medical Center
San Francisco California
Graduated January 1959.

Orthopaedic Specialist Course
Letterman Army Medical Center
San Francisco California
Graduated December 1962.

Clinical Specialist Course

William Beaumont Army Medical
Center
El Paso Texas
Graduated December 1968.

Faculty Development & Admin
Course
Academy of Health Science

Fort Sam Houston Texas
Graduated October 1974.

Military and Civilian Awards:

The Bronze Star Medal

For meritorious achievement in
Ground operations against
Hostile forces Vietnam.

The Meritorious Service Medal

For outstanding service as an
Instructor in the Patient Care
Course Madigan Army Medical
Center Fort Lewis, Washington.

Award of Merit by the National
Authors Registry & Cader
Publishing, for the Chapbook
Titles, "The Sound of Time, and
*"California Mental Health is
Going Down,"* May and June 1993.

Certificates and Licenses:

Licensed Vocational Nurse
California since 1986
Number VN 134546

New York Institute of
Photography
Certificate of Professional
Photography
October 26, 1966 (while
stationed in Japan).

Certified Human Service Worker
ID number c8300848 July 1984

American Society of Orthopaedic
Technologists July 1, 1969.

Community College Limited
Service Credential, Good for life.
Number 356059—issued April
22, 1990

OTHER BOOKS:

The Seduction of Time, et al, Xlibris
Corporation, poetry, 2004.

*Medical Terminology by the
Mnemonic*
Story System, Xlibris
Corporation, 2006.

*Murder in C-Minor, Publish
America, LLL, 2007 (Now
America Star Books). Book
No longer in print.*

What I Do, precursor to this
edition. Xlibris
Corporation, 2008.

The foregoing represents the various parts of my background extending over a period of 48 years. My arrival has more than one point of reference. Nevertheless, if I have to pinpoint any one particular plateau, I would say that the advanced medical specialist course in 1968 was a good one. If we take my arrival to be *teaching*, then we can demonstrate how all the experience up to that date (probably 1974), would show pillar strength or dominance. If you guessed psychointellectual dominance, you would be correct. With that kind of persuasion, one might be a little cold, distant and nerdish. That would be wrong. Although these traits exist, they do not smother me. Vietnam gave me a strong presence of God-fearing along with some experiences about life and death that I shall never forget. With such a past, both the psychointellectual and psychospiritual components of my persona have a healthy existence, leaving the psychochemical part a little behind.

It will not be until 1993 that this neglect of the psychochemical aspect of my persona will be truly realized, and partially corrected.[21] At this time, my arrival was primarily chronological and experiential. In 1974, I began teaching and while this represents true arrival, there would be a great deal more experience and learning before I reached a place where both writing and teaching would meld.

There is a gift of knowledge for all, but that gift is not whole until returned. Duty to others is part of that gift.

---

[21] Coronary quadruple bypass.

CHAPTER NINE

DUTY TO OTHERS

Some say that stating a philosophy, especially in teaching, may give clue to one's underlying biases. Just relating a philosophy may indicate interpretations of life gathered from many sources found inherently interwoven into a discipline, a science, or one's orientation to life, per se. Identifying an existing subjective philosophy, such as one produced by being in a nursing school as an instructor, may reveal a way of doing things common to many schools of nursing, a way of imparting a specific attitude, an ideology placing its catalytic grace upon the force stretched out before humankind, entangled within the moorings of time immemorial. This philosophy then, becomes a byproduct of man's language in action, dedicated to the collective intellect of all that shall follow, founded on the knowledge of the past, and made relevant by the discoveries of today. It is always a process most resistive to the stasis of blind tradition, for all things change. Whatever the fundamental disciplines may have been, the philosophical metamorphosis that results should give clue to certain aspects of nursing that may otherwise go unnoticed, unheeded, or become lost; thereby, leaving each person who has chosen to enter this place to gain their foothold without the stepping stones of wisdom found and used by the many who have gone before.

The nature of man is realized in his unique ability to communicate, to be a time gathering creature, to gather his thoughts and cast them into the sea of knowledge hoping that these many fragmented segments of life's experience will somehow take root, grow and replenish humankind with new data to serve, save and preserve.

To this end, I provide the following creed. It is a personal one. It is a mantra that can be followed by all, not just the nurse, and a way of dealing with reality that has been a viable subjective tool helping me then and today. It is an inner thought for now, a voice for tomorrow, and an instrument of motivation familiar to the minds who teach and for some, a way of life.

MY PERSONAL CREED

Give me courage enough to embrace a vision of the future, keeping my mind elastic to change, always seeking to learn, using my knowledge to aid in the healing of the sick, and mending of the hurt or disabled.

Give me strength enough to stand fast against the eroding force of time, to keep myself healthy, strong, and able to move against our pathogenic foes, disease, misunderstanding, and ignorance.

Give me life enough to finish what I have started, so that I shall not short change anyone in need, and that I may have time to do the best that I can, in search of man and his meaning, here and beyond this mortal vessel.

Give me love enough that I may make peace with my God, as I perceive Him to be, learn to forgive man, but never forget from where I came or where I shall finally go. I am man, transcending the beast, out of woman, a creature with speech, one who has risen above all animal expectations. Though I shall challenge

Nature on all fronts, as man, I must be humble in the shadow of my creator, for in the end of life I shall be held accountable for my deeds done while living, be judged not by man, but by a higher force, and leave behind a heaven or hell for those that follow. In any case, I shall not continue in the form that you now behold.

Give me understanding enough that I shall be able to help those who wander bewildered in mental quandaries, give strength to those who need it in times of trial, and give faith to those who have gone astray in a world of confusing symbols created by man, and his kind.

When all of these gifts have been satisfied, I shall then be whole, for it is in the giving of myself that my true realization becomes actualized, as serving humankind is both my destiny and my end.

Amen

The forgoing written in 1976[22] at the time in my life that great change was happening. I was 43 years old. I was teaching in a military LPN (license vocational nurse) school. I had started teaching in September 1974. This then is the beginning of my self-realization, what my destiny was to become. Happenstance would have it that giving to others through teaching was my way of becoming. To ascend in any pillar one must have experience. Three faculties must exist to assist one in the climb to the acme of pillar success: 1. experience, 2. knowledge, and 3. health. In a way, they all exist together. Experience needs health and knowledge gained along the way. Knowledge is best gotten in a formal sense, which is, going to school or being in an

---

[22] A copy of the letter shown for when the mantra accepted for publication.

apprenticeship. Vocational education may be best for many, as formal education often requires money and aptitude. Probably money is more often an obstacle than aptitude. Nevertheless, I have often assisted those who have less than the needed aptitude into finding their way to achieving a modicum of fulfillment in their chosen field. My gift may be to be able to assist one with their quest in a way that results in some kind of self-achievement. Instructors who are hypercritical and too full of themselves may emotionally cripple students. Every human being has worth; it is our duty to assist with finding a path to that worth.

After teaching for almost six years in the military LPN school, I retired. As disheartening as this was, it was a necessary step.

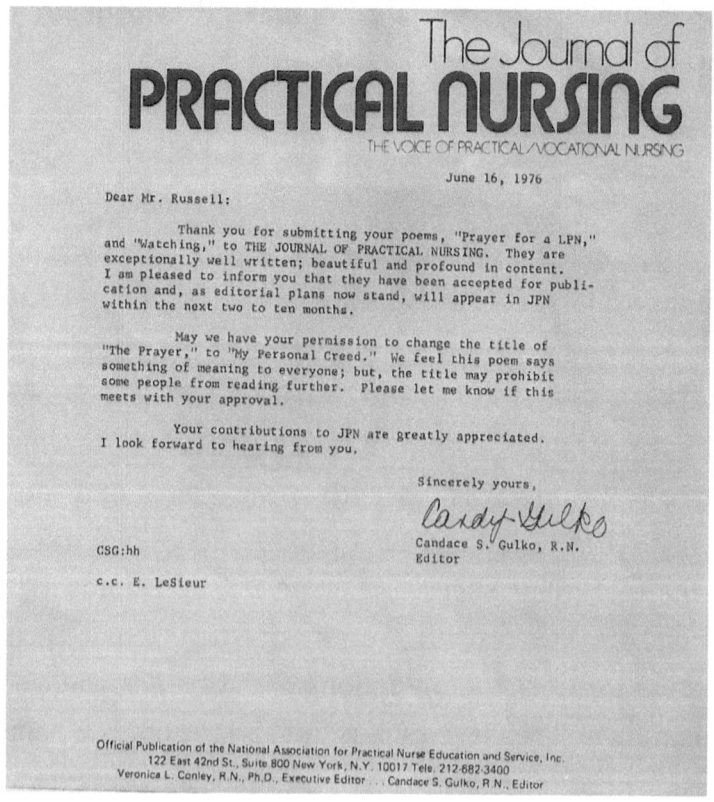

The Journal of
PRACTICAL NURSING
THE VOICE OF PRACTICAL/VOCATIONAL NURSING

June 16, 1976

Dear Mr. Russell:

Thank you for submitting your poems, "Prayer for a LPN," and "Watching," to THE JOURNAL OF PRACTICAL NURSING. They are exceptionally well written; beautiful and profound in content. I am pleased to inform you that they have been accepted for publication and, as editorial plans now stand, will appear in JPN within the next two to ten months.

May we have your permission to change the title of "The Prayer," to "My Personal Creed." We feel this poem says something of meaning to everyone; but, the title may prohibit some people from reading further. Please let me know if this meets with your approval.

Your contributions to JPN are greatly appreciated. I look forward to hearing from you.

Sincerely yours,

Candace S. Gulko, R.N.
Editor

CSG:hh

c.c. E. LeSieur

Official Publication of the National Association for Practical Nurse Education and Service, Inc.
122 East 42nd St., Suite 800 New York, N.Y. 10017 Tele. 212-682-3400
Veronica L. Conley, R.N., Ph.D., Executive Editor . . . Candace S. Gulko, R.N., Editor

CHAPTER TEN

DUTY TO SELF

After spending a very short time at Walla Walla State Penitentiary, in Walla Walla, Washington, and a couple of nursing care centers, I entered employment with Comprehensive Mental Health Center in Tacoma, Washington. As my resume reads, I had about 30 clients. This part of my experience, I am sure, gave me depth in understanding mental health disease as well as issues within the community. In fact, the experience assisted with my hire in my home state, California. After five years working with the mentally ill, I had a new outlook on life. Just having a degree in psychology does not give one experience; coming face-to-face with an ill mind, does.

I remember once when I was about five or so, I had an uncle that had a mural craft studio. He was a photographer back when photography was practically in its infancy. Well, perhaps not that far back, but it was about 1938 or so. His laboratory was huge. There were large tanks and billboard type material strewn throughout this building. My cousin and I would play for hours in this vast place. Today the smell of hypo and developer still bring back those memories. The point in all of this is what he told me one day, "Billy my boy, when you grow up make your hobby your work, it is the best you can do. Do what you love."

Duty to self should be aimed at creating a hobby that can earn you a living. If not a hobby, then find something that you love and make that your life work. Either way you should enjoy what you do. Most often, when you are young it is not possible to do the forgoing. I wanted to be a chemist when I was young. I had a lab and spent many hours working on making explosives, and mixtures of chemicals in preparation for making rockets and the like. It was such fun. There was no pressure from anyone, and I could dream great dreams and build laboratories in the sky. Reality came crashing down when I entered junior college. Back in those days, 1953, they were using slide rules to do computation. Well, you guessed it, I was poor at learning this and the tedium leading into what I considered real chemistry was boring. The truth of the matter was that one must always start at the beginning, not in the middle. I was not mature enough at 20 to realize this, so I changed my major to psychology (sounds like a Freudian slip). After doing poorly with a grade point less than 2.0, I was drafted into the army. This was probably the best thing that could have happened, especially at the age of 21.

The problem with being in the army was that I had little time for duty to self. After two years spent mostly at Fort Ord, California, I received an honorable discharge, 100 dollars, and made the promise that I would join the active reserve unit in my hometown. This I did, at least for the first year. In 1957, I decided to go to Chico College, Chico California. I had been working in the PG&E office in my home town of Willits, California. I was a meter book clerk. This required a little math, legible printing, and taking in payments at the front counter. However, after about a year, I was finding the job pure drudgery, so I decided to go back to college. Off to Chico I went.

College at the age of 24 would be a cinch, right! Wrong. I did not apply myself again, and after only one unsuccessful year and no improvement in grade point I dropped out, got married, and joined the army. This time I had a choice, so I enlisted with a preference in the medical field. After retaking a battery of tests, I had taken them before in 1954 as a draftee; my orders were to attend the Neuropsychiatry Basic Procedure Course given at Letterman General Hospital, Presidio of San Francisco, California. Of course I had to attend basic again, and then general medical training followed by 4 weeks of neuropsychiatric theory at Fort Sam Houston, Texas.

How does this all play into duty to self one might ask? Well, before one can do duty to self, a self has must exist that has depth enough to hold self-worth. One must create a container, a place to hold the substance of being, a realization of self-worth that can be made real. I have known those who walk the land in obscurity, in mental quandaries, lost to the care and love of others. Self-worth comes into being when one gathers the experience for which they have been chosen. It is more than this; it is when the realization comes to them of the reason for their being. Again, it is a place where all three pillars come into play, the psychospiritual, the psychochemical, and the psychointellectual. It is that exclamation, "wow, I know why I am here!" that places one at the plateau of self-esteem. For me it began with the desire to write. The problem with writing at a young age is that you do not have much to say. Having a desire to do does not necessarily equate with ability to do. Before you can do, you must have done, have done the study, have had the experience, and have given the time to your quest. You must pay your dues.

Duty to self is having the discipline to take the time required. Honest toil and study fueled by a quest for understanding/learning. Giving back comes much later.

I spent four years in Neuropsychiatry, five years in Orthopaedics, one year attending an advanced medical (LPN) specialist school, one year in Viet Nam, and finally began teaching at the Clinical Specialist Course at Madigan Army Medical Center, Tacoma, Washington in 1974. I had arrived. My duty to self had ripened.

CHAPTER ELEVEN

THE WORLD OF TEACHING

I was stationed at Fort Lewis, Washington assigned to the 47th Combat Support Hospital (MASH). My assignment to the 47th came right after I returned from Viet Nam in September of 1970. By 1974, I yearned to work again in the medical field proper; the 47th was primarily a training job with no exposure to real patients or hospital wards. To keep our proficiency within our military occupational specialty (MOS) we would rotate periodically working on a ward at Madigan Army Hospital. This was usually no longer than two or three months. Two or three months was not long enough to keep you up to date in your medical specialty, and you were lucky to get one rotation each year, usually around the time that you were required to take your yearly proficiency test. The powers-that-be did not want their clinical specialists to do poorly on the test. Besides that, if you did not do well you would lose your $75.00 proficiency pay. It was time for me to look for a better assignment.

I found out that there was an opening at the advanced medical specialist school Madigan Army Medical Center. I put in the paperwork and on September 2, 1974, I reported to my new duty station. However, I had to attend an Administrative Faculty Development Course given at the Academy of Health Science at Fort Sam Houston, Texas and take the Washington state test for licensed practical nurses before I would be a fully accredited instructor. By the end of 1974, I was ready to start the job of teaching at the Patient Care Specialist Course, Madigan Army Medical Center Tacoma, Washington. However, the journey had just begun. Every journey begins with a first step, as an instructor, that first step is the preparation of behavioral objectives, the DNA of your lesson plan.

Preparing Instructional Objectives

Having just recently graduated from a faculty development course, I was acutely aware of the need to make instruction meaningful, concise, and testable. One method that was in vogue regarded the practice of using instructional objectives from a book by Robert F. Mager.[23] The key word in all of this is *testable*.

In order for anything to be testable, the instructional objectives should follow a threefold presentation:

1. **Performance**. An objective always says what a learner is expected to be able to do; the objective sometimes describes the outcome, the product or result of the doing (behavior)
2. **Condition**. An objective always describes the important conditions under which the performance (behavior) is to occur.
3. **Criterion**. Wherever possible, an objective describes the criterion of acceptable performance by describing how well the learner must perform in order to be considered acceptable, often describing the minimum acceptable

---

[23]   Preparing Instructional Objectives, 1962.

behavior or performance. This threshold allows for assigning a grade in most cases.

Lesson plans were developed with instructional objectives foremost in consideration. Often, behavioral objectives were the key feature of the lesson plan. Some instructors expressed the opinion that all we were teaching were objectives, leaving out important wisdom gathered by those with years of experience in the medical field. The other end of this was the fact that students focused on the objectives to the extent that rich detail in lecture material was not outlined in their notes, just notations referred to by an objective. The example of a written objective within a lesson plan below comes from the ambulatory health rotation that I taught in 1976. You can find the complete lesson plan in the book, "Medical Terminology by the Mnemonic Story System," published by Xlibris, 2006.

I.   Behavioral Objectives:

1.   Briefly discuss or identify the interpersonal or the interaction process as it applies to the following:
    a.   Nursing care philosophy and self,
    b.   Initial patient interview, obtaining a history, and
    c.   Overall screening process, S.O.A.P.ing[24] the patient from start to finish.
2.   Briefly describe or identify the procedure used to perform the examination of the patient with the following: low back pain, cold, flu, and specific trauma to the lower and upper extremities to include at a minimum the following:

---

[24]   Subjective, Objective, Assessment and Plan.

a. Taking a history,

b. Doing the exam,

c. Deciding on an assessment,

d. Plan of action including treatment and follow-up care when necessary, and

e. Final disposition.

Ideally, you would also have a manuscript of the complete instruction, word for word. In the event that you were unable to teach a class, another could do so with the help of the lesson plan and manuscript. I do not know any instructors (today) that have a manuscript. Most instructors just have good notes written on their lesson plan. I have only one such manuscript made when I was attending the faculty development school. I do however have some damn good lesson plans. If you know your subject, you will only need a good lesson plan.

In the six years of teaching within the military clinical specialist course, I grew exponentially as a soldier, as an instructor, and as a person. However, by 1980 I was ready for the next step, returning to civilian life. After 24 years in the military with 1 year in Vietnam and 3 years in Japan, I was ready to find a place and put down some roots. My last year teaching would probably not have been my last year in the army if I had not gotten orders for Germany. After trying to get a relief from orders with no success, I decided that retirement was my best option. In June 1980, I took terminal leave, and finally, said goodbye to a place in life that I shall always miss.

This, however, is not the end of the story. I was 47 with a realization that teaching was my place, my destination, and my resolve; finally, I had arrived. There was still much to learn, but I had been given the opportunity to experience a great deal up to this point. I was honorably discharged into civilian life.

Finding a job teaching so soon after leaving the service was unlikely, but I needed to do something, I was too young to retire fulltime. There were short-term jobs, mostly working with nursing care facilities and mental health services. Finally, I got a job working with a mental health clinic, Comprehensive Mental Health Center, Tacoma, Washington. It was a good job with a great deal to be learned and done. After about two years, I began teaching at a business school in the evening while continuing to work at my day job. I often spent 14 or more hours working each day. The important part of this was that I again taught medical terminology, a subject that I had taught in the military. This time, however, I used a text supplied by the school. In the earlier years, teaching in the military we just put together a course using the books available aided by a good lesson plan. This was mostly just a memorization process often quite difficult for students. The course at the business school consisted of a filmstrip with audio and a book to follow. My primary duty was one of giving the required tests. Any questions from the students were squeezed in at the end of the filmstrip lesson. Not the ideal way to teach even though the author of the book claimed that the average grade for students taking this course was 90 plus percent. As doubtful as I thought that was, I made no changes, nor did I suggest any to the powers-that-be. The students taking the course that I guided averaged about 80 plus percent. It would be much later that I would develop a course of my own, similar but in no way congruent.

Coming Full Circle

I taught my last class at Mendocino College in 2008. From here on out I shall relate what teaching has meant to me and give some examples of style, lesson plans, and a host of data that I hope will pique your interest and lead you into the teaching field allowing you to step free of any land mines; for the teaching terrain can be quite dangerous at times. Today in this, new era of wisdom and caution, our freedom to teach has been eroded by many a fine political movement.

First up comes the separation of church and state. While we have always had certain known rules, few have been as harsh as the ones that exist now. When teaching, one is reminded to be careful not to appear to *preach* one's belief, especially regarding God. I have difficulty with this having spent one year in Vietnam. I often allude to the Almighty, or intimate strongly that faith in medicine is important. On page 96, you can reread *my personal creed*. In my text written for medical terminology, this creed is included. I once had a questionnaire that asked students how they felt about the creed. A student complained to the dean, and I was told to eliminate the questionnaire. I reworded the document, and all was well. I suppose one must also have freedom from religion. Frankly, I worry a lot about a world without God.

Next up for consideration are part time instructors. I had been a part time instructor for twenty years and in all that time was without an ongoing contract. Each semester I received a contract in the mail for the class I usually taught, medical terminology. As a part time employee, I had no permanent status. After teaching for 20 years, I was told that my course would be changed to a distant learning status. Up until that time, medical terminology had been 17 or 18 weeks, a class that would have been better taught in two semesters. Regarding the change to distant learning, I wrote a letter to the dean that I later revised into an article:

Downsizing Education
One Class at a Time

It should be a fundamental right for every student to spend some of their time in a classroom. However, for some subjects the classroom is most important; one such subject is medical terminology. Changing a medical terminology course from 51 hours to 15 hours is like trying to teach someone to swim in a bathtub, you'll get wet, but little else. For medical terminology, distant learning is that bathtub. Changing a course is even more likely to happen to you if you are a part time instructor.

Today many community colleges find it easy to enlist workers part time. Often this means that instructors have no guarantee regarding their ongoing employment. They must succumb to the dictates of circumstance. In the education arena, especially community colleges, this is very much the situation. Part time employees have little to say regarding their class beyond the actual presentation of material. Therefore, if the powers-that-be decide to change the course, delete the course, or alter the way the course is taught, the instructor is bound to comply. Having said this, one can guess what effect this must have on student learning capability when only given the opportunity to take a class by video or another option under the umbrella of distant learning.

Distant learning may bring with it a propensity for one to cheat, parrot back information, and to become an automaton of information, a reflection of the work on the printed page; alas, a bloodless substitute for the reality it purports to portray. Learning should take place in a room with a breathing, feeling person that can provide feedback. After all, isn't that what communication is about, an interchange of ideas between language users capable of sharing feelings, stories, ideas and a host of attributes too long to list. Knowledge cannot exist in a vacuum. Human thought is done best when it is shared with another. Some courses will never lend themselves to a distant learning process.

If we do not take a stand now, when the time comes for our demise, especially as classroom instructors, there will be no one left to stand, the classroom will be bare.

I know that many do not agree with the foregoing, let them. The problem with doing distant learning may be cost. You meet with students for four or five times and get payment the same as your long course. You do the math.

After 20 years, I have developed a great medical terminology course. I do all my own test making and reproducing. The primary text is by an excellent author Davi-Ellen-Chabner. Her book, "The Language of Medicine," is one of the best that I have ever used. It is also one of the most complete, and therefore, often difficult for some students. It is for this reason that two semesters would be better, perhaps a 100 and 200 level class.

The following syllabus is for a 17-week semester.

SYLLABUS

COURSE TITLE: Medical Terminology

CATALOG DESCRIPTION:

The purpose of medical terminology is to furnish an understanding of the need and the reason for the technical language of medicine. To demonstrate how terms come into being, and how they are used. To build a background vocabulary in medical terminology and demonstrate how words are used within the medical arena using the text The Language of Medicine.

CLASS SCHEDULE DESCRIPTION:

Give yourself the power of understanding and using medical terminology. When your doctor says, "The patient must refrain from heterosexual interdigitation." You can say, "Is that so the dactylitis won't become dactylosymphysis?" Enroll in medical terminology today!

STUDENT OUTCOMES:

The student will learn ways to understand, interpret, speak, and write compound medical terms during this course, and:

1. Given a medical term, divide the term into suffix, prefix, and stem; saying out loud, when asked, with correct pronunciation; or, distinguish the meaning by writing a meaning synonym, matching with the correct meaning on a test, or to do so by stating the meaning out loud in class.

2. Given a medical term, use the term in a written or spoken sentence demonstrating an understanding of the term.

3. Answer questions based on text assignments. Complete exercises after each chapter as directed or assigned in class.

COURSE CONTENT AND SCOPE:

A. CHAPTERS:

1. 15 chapters are covered. Chapters not covered may be used for makeup tests and extra assignments per agreement with instructor.

2. There will be one mid-term exam, four or five quizzes, and one final. Adjustments may be made to this schedule

if a lack of time becomes a problem, or there are fewer than 18 weeks for the course.

3. Should a student begin to have difficulty, there will be assistance offered in the Learning Center.[25] In addition, makeup tests will be available in the Learning Center. An alternate test can be given to assist a student with the possibility of a passing grade. To qualify for makeup testing the grade must be a failing grade, i.e. 59% or lower. The makeup test will allow for a grade no higher than 69%; or, the two test scores averaged together, whichever is highest.

B.   LECTURE INFORMATION BY TOPIC:

1. Orthopaedics,
2. Neuropsychiatry,
3. General Surgical/Anatomical descriptions (if time allows),
4. Cardiology (text chapter 11), and
5. Unannounced.

C.   READING ASSIGNMENTS:

Students are required to read/study chapters as assigned in text as well as any handouts that may be given to them. Assigned library reading or Learning Center work may be used to substitute for lost time.

---

[25]   Testing at Mendocino Community College by this center has been changed, check with your instructor.

D. WRITING ASSIGNMENTS:

Substantial writing assignments in this course are not necessary as the primary way to respond is in the nature of a written form; as in, quizzes, tests, and makeup work.

E. OUT OF CLASSROOM ASSIGNMENTS/STUDY:

Two (2) hours of study outside of class for each hour in class is advised. The reading assignments alone should comprise at least two (2) hours. More when there are several chapters involved. Fifteen (15) chapters allowing for an average time of two (2) hours for each should give each student enough hours to qualify for 50% of the two (2) hours required.

F. ASSIGNMENTS THAT DEMONSTRATE CRITICAL THINKING:

Students will demonstrate the ability to think critically by performing the following tasks:

1. Given a compound medical word, divide into suffix, prefix, and stem, and when asked, say the meaning out loud or write a meaning synonym on a test, or match the word with its correct meaning, or to do so in class by stating the meaning out loud after correct pronunciation of the word and/or giving a definition or meaning on a written test.

2. Given a medical term, use the term/word in a written or spoken sentence demonstrating an understanding of the meaning of the term/word by creating a new sentence using the term/word. Or, by matching, identifying, or selecting a meaning of a medical term/word on a written test.

3. Follow all behavioral objectives for each chapter and complete exercises as directed.

G. METHOD OF INSTRUCTION:

Lecture with discussion in class of the exercises taken from text. Additional lectures as time allows. Examinations taken from text will be in the format that is shown in text. If time allows, one film on orthopaedics. Handouts as needed, especially those that compliment the text, taken from text or other periodicals, and are shown as transparencies.

For students having difficulty, an alternate method of study is available. See instructor. Using the book, "*Medical Terminology by the Mnemonic Story System,*" found in the Learning Center, an alternate method may be applied and tested. Using the alternate system of study will allow for the highest grade of 69%, especially for those that have failed a test or quiz. *Attention*: the method just described is not a required method; it is only suggested for those having difficulty with the primary text. If after reviewing the book in the Learning Center, you wish to purchase a copy, see the instructor, a copy can be ordered; or, check the college bookstore.

H. METHOD OF EVALUATION:

A. Mid-term examination = 25% of total grade.

B. Five quizzes = 25% of total grade.

C. Final examination = 50% of total grade.

There is extra credit available for those having difficulty. In addition, there is makeup testing available at the Learning Center. Examinations will be placed in the Learning Center on the day of the test, and will be left there until all who have missed have taken them or until the end of the thirteenth week. No makeup work will be accepted after the fourteenth week. Any examination not done by the fourteenth week will be graded as a zero. See section questions often asked regarding bonus points.

I. **TEXT**: *The Language of Medicine*, Davi-Ellen Chabner, B.A., M.A.T., seventh edition, W.B. Saunders Company.

J. CAUSE FOR DROPPING FROM CLASS:

Students will be dropped from this class if there is a waiting list, and they do not come on the first meeting without appropriate notification. A student may be dropped at any time during the course if they miss three days, or more, at the instructor's discretion.

Study Guide

Fall Mid-Term	Spring Mid-Term	Final
Page 15, 16	Page 14	Chapters 1, 2, 3, & 4
Page 19, 47	Page 17	Chapters 5,9, & 10
Page 61, 63	Page 61, 63	Chapters 11,12, &15
Page 92, 95	Page 93, 96	Chapters 17, 20, 21, & 22
Page 125, 130	Page 125, 126	
Page 171, 237	Page 171, 174	
Page 240	Page 237, 240, 242, 243	
Page 323	Page 323, 325	
Page 367	Page 367, 370	

MEDICAL TERMINOLOGY WEEKLY SCHEDULE
For the text, "The Language of Medicine"

WEEK: **DESCRIPTION:**

1. _____   Introduction (Orientation)
Read chapter one before class
Exercises explained

2. _____   **Read chapter two before class**
Word building
Exercises in text

3. _____   **Read chapter three before class**
Exercises in text

4.   _____   **Read chapter four before class**

Exercises in text

5.   _____   **Read chapter five on digestion system (Before class)**

Quiz number one (1) Chapter 1-4 (40 minutes)

Exercises in text

6.   _____   **Read chapter seven, the urinary system (Before class)**

Exercises in text

7.   _____   **Read chapter nine, male reproduction system (Before class)**

Discussion & exercises in text

8.   _____   **Read chapter ten, nervous system, before class**

Quiz number two (2) on chapter nine, male Reproductive system

Exercises in text

9.   _____   Mid-Term Test

You may leave after test.

10.   _____   **Read chapter eleven, cardiovascular system (Before class)**

Exercises in text

11.   _____   **Quiz number three (3) cardiovascular system**

Read chapter twelve, respiratory system (Before class)

Exercises in text

12. _____ **Read chapter fifteen, musculoskeletal system (Before class)**

Exercises in text, lecture with handout

13. _____ **Quiz number four (4), musculoskeletal system**

Read chapter seventeen, sense organs (Before class) exercises in text

14. _____ **Read chapter twenty before class, Radiology and Nuclear Medicine.** Exercises, discussion.

15. _____ **Read chapters 21 & 22 before class**

Text exercises & discussion, handout

16. _____ **Quiz number five (5) on psychiatry 1st hour**

Last two hours guest speaker on dental, bring questions

From handout booklet

17. _____ **Final examination (usually from 5 to 7 pm)**

Chapters not covered can be used for extra credit or for additional credit. When used for additional credit, the project must be finished before the 14th week.

Handouts Given As Part of Introduction to Class

The Teacher Talks
To The Student

I am not all knowing. If I lead you to believe that I am, then, I am a fool. There may be times when it seems that this is so, but this is because I have been down this road before; at best, I can only point out the highlights to you. Your vision is young and new and mine is older, tinted with shades of time and experience. Though you may learn from me, understand that you learn much through the wide eyes of youth and much, much more from each other. Your questions will help to make you rich in the knowledge mined from the territory you shall travel. I only hope that God will grant me the patience, time and the gift of giving and sharing with you my stored knowledge and experience in an unselfish manner; for in this sharing we shall both grow. I may very well learn a great deal more from you than you from me, for you are many and I am but one.

I see the territory before us with the eyes of experience shaded from the glitter of youth's haste. I have not lost the excitement in viewing the unfolding(s) before us. I still enjoy the rediscovery of each new fact seen anew through your eyes, I share a vicarious pleasure in each new search for truth, each new pain of growing, and wisdom reclaimed.

I have enough love for my work, for my ideals and for you that given the opportunity I will share all within my limits. However, remember, I am only one, so forgive me if I seem shallow at times, or spent, or even used, I may be. I admire honesty, ambition, and self-actualization, but hold sacred our relationship. For, we may indeed share a oneness as rare as the feeling of love. We do need each other, and we shall achieve a greatness that few can profess if we can shed the outer garments of distrust that can tend to repel us, one from the other. Our purpose here is evident, and though we are teacher and pupil, we share in a creation of time gathering, a destiny that shall make us immortal.

––––––––––––––––––––––

An Introduction to Medical Terminology
[by way of: Med-Term by the Mnemonic Story System]
Used in the 17 week course with *The Language of Medicine*[26]

The following questions are from the book in the Learning Center with the title, "Medical Terminology by the Mnemonic Story System." Ref.: "An Introduction to Ambulatory Health Care Philosophy", appendix—page 125. The assignment is optional for bonus points.

These are bonus questions. If you complete by 2nd week = 20 points; 4th week 15 points; 6th week 10 points; and, 8th week 5 points.

1. In the author's opinion, what constitutes the necessary thinking for one to be in nursing?

    _____

    _____

    _____

2. In establishing common verbal bonds, what is the author's opinion of one who cannot demonstrate that they care in the process of gathering information from a client?

    _____

    _____

    _____

---

[26] *The Language of Medicine,* Chabner, Davi-Ellen, B.A., M.A.T., Saunders, 7th edition, 2004. When this was the primary text for a 17-week course and *Med-Term by the Mnemonic Story System* was a reference text.

3. Name three causes of low back pain.

_____

_____

_____

4. In your opinion, how thorough is the list "guide to physical exam" for *eliciting possible disc disease?* (Written before popular use of MRI)

_____

_____

_____

5. What do you think, "to designate one as a psychosomatic is for the diagnostically destitute," means?

_____

_____

_____

6. Was there anything that stood out, got your attention?

_____

_____

_____

7. Did you look at any of the rest of the book? If so, what do you think of it?

_____

_____

_____

Questions Often Asked

Q-1.   What happens if I am unable to complete the course?

A-1   You will be given an incomplete. You then have about one year to make up the work missed. If you do not you may get a failure, or a grade equal to work completed.

Q-2   How can I make up a test/quiz that I have missed?

A-2   All test/quizzes are placed in the learning center on the day of the test.
       You usually[27] have one week to take them. If you do not your grade will be a zero. Makeup work can be substituted for missed tests/quizzes.

Q-3   Can I make up a failure?

A-3   You can retake the test or quiz. A retake allows for a grade no higher than 69%, or the average between the two tests, whichever is higher?

Q-4   How are bonus points scored?

A-4   Bonus points on quizzes count as one point. If after you have completed all quizzes and you have an excess number, these can be applied to the lowest quiz score only once. After you finish the quizzes and have an excess number of points but do not need them, as all your quizzes are at least 90%, the quiz points can be divided by 4 and

---

[27]   All work, including makeup of quizzes or tests, has to be done by the fourteenth week. However, it is always best to do any such work as soon as possible. (This option no longer available, 2014).

used against a low mid-term score (below 70%). Mid-term bonus points can be used against the final, x 0.42.

Q-5 Is there any outside work that one can do for extra credit.

A-5 Yes, an assignment taken from the book. "Medical Terminology by the Mnemonic Story System," See page 9. If you do not do this assignment you lose the possibility of gaining the bonus points.

Q-6 When is the latest that one can finish any work not done?

A-6 All work and makeup tests must be done by the 14th week, no exceptions.

Q-7 How many days can I miss without a penalty?

A-7 After 3 days, one can be dropped from the course. However, if there is a medical reason, or a reason of circumstance, one may be given a waiver, and allowed to continue. Whatever the reason, the instructor should be notified. If one misses more than two quizzes and/or the mid-term, this may be cause for failure.

Q-8 When is the final, and what time does it start?

A-8 The final exam is given on the last day of class. If the class is a 5:30 to 8:30pm class, the final will be given from five to 7pm. Do not come at 5:30 as you will be losing one half hour.

Q-9 Is there a way to contact you about assignments and to let you know when a class will be missed?

A-9 E-mail: MnemonicBooks@aol.com, or phone # 463-0892.

Q-10 Are there any special considerations for classroom etiquette that you require?

A-10 Several. I require people to not talk or visit with their friends during class. To do so is most impolite. If I have to ask one person more than twice, I may then ask that person to leave for that class. I prefer that men do not wear hats in the class. No food or drink is allowed by school policy. Water may be allowed, if there is a cap on the bottle that can be used to keep the water from spilling when not in use. While difficult to enforce, please be considerate of others when wearing perfume and/or shaving lotion for men. Strong scents may set off allergies in others, be cautious. Summertime brings excessive perspiration, be considerate.

Cautionary Note:

Medical terminology is a language that often describes body functions and physiology. Using pee pee and poo poo is not going to make it; we must use the words as they appear within the text. Therefore, if you wish not to hear these Latin and Greek equivalents to these functions, you may be in the wrong course

BIBLIOGRAPHY

(Included for student use)

Chabner, Davi-Ellen. *"The Language of Medicine."* W.B. Saunders Company. 2004, 7th edition.

Dorland's Illustrated Medical Dictionary. W.B. Saunders Company. 1981, 26th edition.

Ehrilch, Ann. *"Medical Terminology for the Health Professionals."* Delmar Publishers. 1997, 3rd edition.

Glazier, Teresa Ferster. *"The Least You Should Know about Vocabulary Building Word Roots."* Holt, Rhinehart & Winston, Inc. 1990, 3rd edition.

Harned, J.E. *"Medical Terminology Made Easy."* Physician's Record Company. 1968, 2nd edition.

Russell, William J. *"Medical Terminology by the Mnemonic Story System."* Mnemonic Publishers, Ukiah, CA 95482, 2006, 1st edition, Xlibris Corporation (Look for it in the college bookstore)

Skinner, Henry Alan. *"The Origin of Medical Terms."* The Williams & Wilkins Company. 1949, 1st edition.

Tabers Cyclopedic Medical Dictionary. F.A. Davis Company. 2001, 19th edition.

It should be the responsibility of anyone having the duty to teach to be aware of his or her motivation, need, desire, or reason for doing so. A firm platform of conviction may not be enough. Each of us has an internal vision of how we think the world is. Having an awareness of that internal view and the way it fits with the true reality of existence gives one a beginning for the quest for truth. How one lives one's life, is as important as what one believes, for the two are often inseparable (At this point my personal creed is inserted, page ___)

In the late summer of 2006, I was informed that my medical terminology class would be changed to a distant learning style. I was also told that eventually my class would become an online course. I thought that I would try the online course when it came time, hoping that it would be several years before that happened.

While teaching my last regular class in the fall of 2006, I began filming the part of the class that used flashcards based on the book, *Medical Terminology by the Mnemonic Story System*. I did the filming during an actual class. I also had given to the dean of instruction a well-written lesson plan describing the preparation for the class.[28] This plan was both a description and a permission to do. The following spring the first class began. The following is the syllabus used for the class.

---

[28]   See endnote number 4 for this book.

Syllabus for a distant learning course

SYLLABUS

SUBJECT AREA AND COURSE NUMBER _____

COURSE TITLE: Medical Terminology (Distant Learning)

CATALOG DESCRIPTION:

To furnish an understanding of the need and reason for the technical language of medicine, and to demonstrate how terms come into being, how they are used and formed. To build a background vocabulary in medical terminology and demonstrate a word building system using mnemonic (memory) devices or phrases that make it easier for the user to understand and remember a growing medical terminology.

CLASS SCHEDULE DESCRIPTION:

Give yourself the power of understanding and using medical terminology. When your doctor says, "the patient must refrain from heterosexual interdigitation." You can say, "Is that so the dactylitis won't become dactylosymphysis?" Enroll in medical terminology today!

STUDENT OUTCOMES/OBJECTIVES:

The student will learn ways to understand, divide the term into suffix, prefix, speak, and write complex (compound) medical terms, and:

1. Given a medical term, divide the term into suffix, prefix, and stem saying aloud with correct pronunciation, or distinguish the meaning by writing a meaning synonym on a test, or by stating the meaning aloud in class.

2. Given a medical term use the term/word in a written or spoken sentence demonstrating an understanding of the term/word.

COURSE CONTENT AND SCOPE:

A. CHAPTERS

1. Chapter 1 will be covered during orientation.

2. Chapters 2 through 11 will be covered by CD found in the learning center. Also, can be purchased at the bookstore.

3. Chapter 12 is a read only chapter; it will not be covered by a CD.

B. LECTURE INFORMATION WITH TOPICS:

Lectures included in the videos

1. Orthopaedic conditions,

2. Pharmacology, and

3. Neuropsychiatry (included with a handout).

C. READING ASSIGNMENTS:

Students are required to read all chapters 1 thru 12. Students are required to read handouts and be familiar with the appendices of the book.

D. WRITING ASSIGNMENTS:

In 500 words, but not less than 350 words, write an essay that relates to the use of medical terminology in your life. The essay is due by the third meeting. A student may select to write an additional essay on any subject relating to the use of medical terminology. The instructor must approve these assignments before written, and an essay may accrue points to assist with a test grade.

E. OUT OF CLASSROOM ASSIGNMENTS/STUDY:

Viewing of the videos and reading should cause one to accumulate at least 2 hours for each chapter. Do the practice exercises in the book.

F. ASSIGNMENTS THAT DEMONSTRATE CRITICAL THINKING:

Students will demonstrate the ability to think critically by performing the following tasks.

1. Given a compound medical word, divide into suffix, prefix and stem, saying the meaning aloud or write a meaning synonym on a test; or to do so in class by stating the meaning aloud after correct pronunciation of the compound medical word.

2. When given a medical term, use the term in a written or spoken sentence demonstrating an understanding of the meaning of the term by creating a new sentence using the term.

3. When given a medical term on a test write the element meaning in lay terms. Example: For cardio-, give the response heart.

4. Identify word elements when introduced in a written paragraph of association/images with mnemonic device taken from lessons in a story format by defining the element.

Example: The card was the ace of hearts. Mnemonic device is card. The medical term is cardio-. The meaning is heart. On a story test, you would be looking for the medical element. Review the practical exercise in the story test, (Beauty and the Ace). Read the story and see if you can figure out the medical word elements referred to in the story. There are eight.

G.   METHOD OF INSTRUCTION:

The student will view the 10 videos chapters 2 through 11. Some lecture format is included within the video format. Classroom time allowed is 15 hours as one meeting of 3 hours each month. The first 3 hours will be an orientation. Meetings 2 through 4 will be designated for 2-hour tests with a minimal of lecture/discussion depending on how long it takes all students to complete the test. Usually this will be no longer than 2 hours. The last meeting is for the final exam.

H. METHODS OF EVALUATION:

Three 100 element tests = 40% of grade and 1 final = 50% of the grade. Additional assigned work for 10% of the grade. Or, 50% for 3 tests and 50% for 1 final, whichever is most appropriate for the student.

Grades: D = 60 to 69%; C = 70 to 79%; B = 80 to 89%; and, A = 90 to 100%.

I.   **TEXT:** Medical Terminology by the Mnemonic Story System, William J. Russell, first edition, 2006, Xlibris Corporation, www.Xlibris.com

J. REPEATABLE FOR CREDIT:

This course teaches a basic vocabulary in medical terminology. It is possible that there will be students that want to repeat this course as a refresher only. To do so, one would have to check with the admission and records department.

SCHEDULE FOR CLASSROOM AND STUDY

1. _____ Orientation
Review chapter 1 in class

2. _____ Review video chapters 2 and 3

3. _____ Review video chapter 4

4. _____ Review video chapter 5

5. _____ Test Number 1 (ab—to gingiv-)
Discussion/Lecture if time permits

6. _____ Review video chapters 5 and 6

7. _____ Review video chapter 7

8. _____ Review video chapter 8

9. _____ Test Number 2 (glom—to—penia)
Discussion/Lecture if time permits

10. _____ Review video chapter 9

11. _____ Review video chapter 10

12. _____ Review video chapter 11

13. _____ Study for test number 3

14. _____ Test Number 3 (pep—to vulse-)
Discussion/Lecture if time permits

15. _____ Review ad lib
Study for final
Research projects

16. _____ Review ad lib
Study for final
Research projects

17. _____ Final Exam
You may leave after test

Example of the handout used for Neuropsychiatry lecture

EVALUATION OF MENTAL HEALTH
THROUGH THE PATHOS OF SCHIZOPHRENIA

They say California Mental Health is burning,
From dust we came, ashes to ashes,
They say Mental Health will have to crash;
Crash and burn before anyone will care.

State audit virus, self-impelled,
Burn too, please do;
Your quest to strangle your host,
Fails safe in fire white-hot.

Phoenix rising in new form
I doubt you worry too much,
Those who fell with you
Are barely warm—
But oh, how they felt the fiery storm!

The California mental health system is in the throes of change. Ever since the system dumped clients on the streets in the 1970s, there has been a promise of help that did not quite make it. Instead, the cost containment bug bit deeply into the already depleted system of mental health under the watchful eye of federally mandated programs. The California mental health system is a system going down, now in the 21st century, and back then in the late 1990s.

Why the system needs change:

1. Clients and family members are telling us that what we have been doing is not working; today, it is still not working, all played on deaf ears.

2. The marketplace of public and private health services, including mental health, has changed to require some form of cost containment;

3. Because of funding shifts and an overall paucity of fiscal resources, counties are increasingly aware of their financial "risk" when client outcomes are not achieved, or a client dies while in criminal custody;

4. There is competition now for the Medi-Cal mental health dollar. If counties are to continue to be the primary provider of public mental health services, they will have to change to produce outcomes and "customer" satisfaction; and,

5. Education of the public concerning the three most misunderstood mental health diseases: schizophrenia, bipolar illness, and major depression.

If we look at only one mental health related disease, that disease being schizophrenia, and explore the process briefly using the tool called Quality Assurance, we may be given a modicum of insight; perhaps, even understanding.

Defining Schizophrenia:

Schizophrenia comes to us from the Greek meaning split mind; a name for *split personality* coined by Eugen Bleuler as an alternative for dementia praecox. It appears in his book "Textbook of Psychology." The term has been used generally to mean dementia praecox, but it is only one form of this condition. Dementia praecox, as such, has become an obsolete term for schizophrenia; although, with our present understanding of schizophrenia, the concept of dementia, per se, may not have been far afield. However, dementia is regarded as an organic mental syndrome or disorder. Where the two definitions touch is in the definition of the word organic (organic has to do with brain chemistry and relates to the many necessary chemicals needed for the brain to function neuro-electrically) as it relates to schizophrenia and dementia. Schizophrenia is an organic brain disease. Dementia is also an organic brain disease, but lacks the organization of delusions and hallucinations. Dementia has primarily to do with short term and long term memory, impaired judgment, other disturbances of higher cortical function such as aphasia (disorder of language), apraxia (inability to carry out motor activities despite intact sensory function), and personality change. Our understanding of schizophrenia today has produced a chasm between what is dementia and what is schizophrenia.

Schizophrenia [**Gr.** phren, mind] as a word, does indeed mean *split mind*. What the meaning should relate is that this is a brain disease, which causes one's thinking process to be split from reality in some way. As a diagnosis schizophrenia presents with *delusions* (false beliefs); *prominent hallucinations* (voices in one's head that no one else can hear, or visual images that no other can see); *incoherence or marked loosening of associations* (loss of logical, connected thinking where one thought may not connect with another); *catatonic behavior* (lead pipe flexibility, where one can stand for hours without moving while allowing extremities to be moved after which they will remain where moved); *flat or grossly inappropriate affect* (no expression at all, or smile while telling one that their father died). The foregoing is a psychotic process, and therefore, schizophrenia, as such, is a psychosis rather than a neurosis.

Although there is no single symptom that is only found in schizophrenia, several are found very uncommonly in diseases other than schizophrenia. Kurt Schneider, a German psychiatrist, proposed a list of symptoms he called *first rank* symptoms, meaning that when one or more of them are present they point strongly toward schizophrenia as a diagnosis. This list is:

1. Auditory hallucinations in which the voices speak to ones thoughts aloud.
2. Auditory hallucinations with two voices arguing.
3. Auditory hallucinations with voices commenting on ones actions.
4. Hallucinations of touch when the bodily sensation is imposed by some external agency.
5. Withdrawal of thoughts from one's mind.
6. Insertion of thoughts into one's mind by others.
7. Believing one's thoughts are being broadcast to others, as by radio or television.

8. Insertion by others of feelings into one's mind.
9. Insertion by others of irresistible impulses into one's mind.
10. Feelings that one's action are under the control of others, like an automaton.
11. Delusions of perception, as when one is certain that a normal remark has secret meaning.

While the foregoing represents symptoms commonly used in European countries, grounds for diagnosis in the United States are less likely to use this list. American psychiatry took a major step in 1980 when it adopted a revised system of diagnosis and nomenclature and issued it in a third edition of the Diagnostic and Statistical Manual of Mental Disorders, usually referred as DSM-III, and today in the 1990s as the DSM-IV, and all changes today in the year 2014.

Somewhere between the definition of schizophrenia and our understanding of the reality exists the actuality. Schizophrenia has carried the metaphor of being the *virus* of psychiatry. When all attempts at understanding a mental aberration failed, schizophrenia often became the label. Today, with new understanding, that label has specificity and treatment should be more than palliative, but often it is not. Our next observation should be of the language used to give treatment. This plan called quite properly, the treatment plan.

Treatment Planning Under Traditional Quality Assurance:

Historically, it has been that you do an intake, then follow with a diagnosis that leads to treatment goals that you, the therapist, devise with the clients help, or input. This system called the *problem oriented medical record* (POMR), dealt with the laborious recording of signs and symptoms as well as the problems created by them. Each of the problems had to relate to medical necessity, and each had to be addressed in the treatment plan by number. As the system developed, it was necessary to devise a way to know when the treatment plan directives had been accomplished. Sometime in the 1970s (probably influenced by the educational system), the concept of treatment objectives came to be used. Treatment objectives were described in behavioral terms. Traditional therapy gave way to descriptions of behavioral outcomes that needed to be accomplished in specific periods approved by quality assurance committees. Federal and State mandated programs began to tighten the grip on moneys and this constriction began to make itself apparent in the funds available to the mental health clinics.

With the advent of new constrictions came new language and traditional psychotherapy (especially for schizophrenia), should have died and been reborn in new form. This did not quite happen. Quality assurance in the 1980s tried to do both; it tried to meet the new precepts of treatment while maintaining the old theoretical tenets of psychotherapy. This gave rise to a dichotomy that still pervades the mental health system today.

Schizophrenia has been thought, in the past, to be either organic or functional. Traditional psychotherapy would deal with the idea that insight oriented therapy would help by bringing the client in touch with causes that were related to outside influences, and therefore functional, while those who supported the organic premise of brain disease would stabilize the client with medications. Others would use both techniques using medication first and then when the client was stable, provide therapy as an adjunct; in some cases, this was not in the form of insight oriented therapy per se, but a form of cognitive therapy technique combined with assisting the client with activities of daily living with emphasis on lodging, food, and self care.

Treatment planning became a process of utilizing both medication and psychotherapeutic technique. The primary difficulty with this made itself seen in the diverse format used in both progress notes and treatment plan format. With such diversity in format and description, it soon became evident that no two counties did anything alike. Each county quality assurance coordinator was charged with the duty to provide, with the assistance of various committees, and guidelines based on State mandated programs, proof of medical necessity to assure that each case treated qualified for reimbursement. With so many different ways of doing things, there were fertile grounds for audit exceptions and the recoupment of the federal share of funding. It was obvious that some kind of change was needed.

Because there was now no money for the long treatment found in most traditional forms of psychotherapy, another approach seemed evident. In late 1989, the California department of mental health issued a policy letter with the subject title: Case management services. Each of the 58 counties were required to create policy based on this letter to be submitted for approval, and one that would have to be validated by an audit at some later date. Case management is almost a quantum leap from traditional therapy, providing services that have to do with Evaluation, Plan Development, Emergency Intervention, Placement Services, Assistance in Daily Living, and Consultation. These services required a different approach in thinking for therapists who had been used to a model primarily designed to intervene psychotherapeutically. The focus of *curing* the malady became less important and the idea of *containment* and the reduction of recidivism more to the forefront. Case management seemed to offer more for less. You could now use mental health workers who were long on experience, but short on the postgraduate degrees needed in traditional mental health care, to be case managers; so long as there was a mental health professional that would oversee their work and provide guidance.

The immediate change was one of focus. Instead of looking primarily at psychopathology, client care in the community was addressed. The quality of care for chronically ill schizophrenics improved, it seemed, for the care had stepped into the lives of the clients beyond the walls of the mental health clinic and into their lives on the streets. It was obvious to any outsider that something had changed. Case management was an active process and did not have the passive constraints of the so-called psychotherapeutic environment within the hallowed walls of the mental health clinic. In a word, it was personal.

Case management, while not a new concept, may be the precursor on the way to a better system of care. This direction of treatment may be a swing back through time. Mental health professionals may have to hit the streets. An influx of technicians may arrive on the scene to assist the already overworked clinicians in the endless battle against the ever increasing sea of homeless and mentally ill walking our promised land; a land that is as much theirs as ours. When the state of California dumped financial responsibility on the counties for care of the mentally ill, a situation already sad became worse. When administrative personnel make medical decisions, clients suffer.

What ever the future holds, it is sure to bring changes in how quality assurance coordinators perform their jobs. The fact of cost containment is present today and will be tomorrow. Questions that you and I should ask are, "Will mental health clinicians continue to do more with less? Will the streets become the camping ground for an ever-increasing number of mentally ill? Will health care for the mentally ill in this 21st century be something we as citizens can be proud to behold? You can judge a country by how it takes care of the education of the young, the medical care of the aged, and those who walk the streets in mental quandaries. How must we be judged today? Tomorrow? Are we indeed our brothers' keeper, or just onlookers, ones who walk the plank of destiny, blindfolded to the reality of now, you tell me!

In the foregoing, the two syllabi represent the difference between 51 hours of instruction and 15 hours. It should be easy to see why I wrote the article on distant learning. An example of a lesson plan for the neuropsychiatric portion of the class is next. It can be used for both a long class and a distant learning class. Although, with the constriction of time, I doubt that it would work when you only have 15 hours of classroom time.

Lesson Planning

The lesson plan is your guide to teaching. There is no way that anyone can remember verbatim more than a mere grasp of any subject. Using an abbreviated format saves time, aids memory, and keeps one from going astray. Written well, a lesson plan can serve as a handout, putting in blank spaces for the student to fill in. Even if wandering is your style, having a lesson plan allows you to come back to your point of departure; the only thing lost may be time. By the way, I believe that richness in teaching style can be accredited, in part, to one's ability to tell stories and relate strong metaphors based on experience. Students have often told me that my stories, experiences, and metaphors are what make the class interesting.

An example of a lesson plan follows:

I. Introduction:

A. Schizophrenic Places

> Let us gather up some sleepless nights
> With paranoid visitations in hasty flights
> Found in schizophrenic places
> Complete with haunted faces
> Demonic dungeons in tissue abide
> On faceless neurons of minds tongue-tied

Where delusions play upon a tortured soul
Ranting their soundless rasp of malcontent
While therapies pointlessly interrogate
To understand a chemistry with words
Where words—at best—collide with words
While therapies insult and insinuate
So long as disease must here reside
That long their words not reach inside

B. Objectives: As stated in the book <u>The Language of Medicine,</u> chapter twenty-two.

C. Class Procedure and Lesson Tie-in: The primary lesson will concern the three major mental illnesses: schizophrenia, major depression, and bipolar disorder.

II. Explanation:

A. Show the DSM-IV (or most recent issue)

B. Relate a little about each:

1. Psychiatrist (4 years med school) and then a varying number of years learning their craft.

2. Psychoanalyst (3 to 5 years learning techniques in the process of psychoanalysis.

3. Psychologist (minimum of a master's degree) in one of several specialties.

C. Tests to Evaluate Mental Health:

1. Wechsler Adult Intelligence Scale

2. Stanford-Binet Intelligence Scale

3. Thematic Apperception Test (TAT) also, *tell a tale*. This technique is known as a projective test. Another example is the Rorschach test.

D. Clinical Symptoms:

1.	Amnesia	9.	Dysphoria
2.	Anxiety	10.	Euphoria
3.	Apathy	11.	Hallucination
4.	Autism	12.	Labile
5.	Compulsion	13.	Mania
6.	Conversion	14.	Mutism
7.	Delusion	15.	Obsession
8.	Dissociation	16.	Paranoia

E. Freudian Interpretation of a reality thought to be.

1. Id, a representation of unconscious instincts and psychic energy present at birth and represents the child.

2. Ego, mediates between the demands of the id and the realities of the external world. (Compare with adult and self) The ego is the central control or decider system of the personality and is said to operate in terms of the reality principle.

3. Superego, the outgrowth of learning the taboos and moral values of society. In essence, the superego is what we refer to as the conscience, and is concerned with good, bad, right, and wrong. (Compare with parent)

The primary weaknesses in many of Freud's axiomatic conclusions about man may have been his lack of scientific method. Many of his case studies were based on but one person, a process that led him to much introspection. However, some say that from such a great intellect, a little introspection may reveal much. I am not so sure.

The following is an observation that I made some years ago while watching Star Trek. It is given to be used as an anecdotal relief when you notice that student attention span is beginning to wander.

TREK THERAPY

Wouldn't it be great if just watching a TV program gave you the equivalent of one hour of therapy, and this therapy has provided you with an aftermath of well being? Made you feel better each time you watched the program. Well, that may not be too far from actuality.

In the 1960s there was a personality theory called transactional analysis. Developed initially by a psychiatrist, Eric Berne (1961, 1964), and popularized by Thomas Harris (1969) a psychiatrist. Transactional analysis is essentially a procedure for evaluating interactions between people regarding three ego states: child, adult, and parent. An individual is seen as having potentials in all three of these ego states, but in any particular situation with another person, he may be found usually in one of those states. Thus, John may be a child in relationship to his wife, dealing with her symbolically as though she was his mother; and, with his friends, he may be a parent taking a supervisory role.

If we look at only the implication that these three ego states represent; the parent, one who cares and is in charge; the adult, one who is logical, and often sees things as black and white; and the child, who is playful, and can be quite illogical at times, we can see endless combinations as the three states interact.

An example of the process has to do with the TV program Star Trek. Consider the three ego states as individuals. James Kirk represents our parent figure. Mr. Spock plays the adult, and the Child is Dr. "Bones" McCoy. In each episode, these three characters interact while solving some problem of space, time, or state of being. As we watch these three personalities interact, we find our self-drawn in to the situation at hand. As the play comes to a climax, we too feel the situation, by vicarious identification. Finally, when all has been solved, completed, and the end is before us, we feel whole. In the process of watching, we have drawn these three parts of our own self together. And for the moment, we are whole. We feel good, at least, until we get another fix with the next episode.

Okay, back to the outline.

III. Disorders:

    A. Anxiety Disorders

    B. Delirium and Dementia

    C. Dissociative Disorders

    D. Eating Disorders

    E. Mood Disorders

          1. Bipolar I and II

          2. Cyclothymic

          3. Dysthymia

          4. Major Depression

    F. Personality Disorders

          1. Antisocial

          2. Borderline

          3. Histrionic

          4. Narcissistic

          5. Paranoid

          6. Schizoid

    G. Schizophrenia (handout)

    H. Sexual and Gender Identity Disorders

          1. Exhibitionism

          2. Fetishism

          3. Pedophilia

          4. Sexual Masochism

          5. Sexual Sadism

6. Transvestic Fetishism
7. Voyeurism

I. Somatoform Disorders
1. Hypochondriasis
2. Conversion Disorder

IV. Therapeutic Intervention

A. Psychotherapy
1. Behavior therapy
2. Family therapy
3. Group therapy
4. Hypnosis
5. Psychoanalysis
6. Sex therapy

B. Eclectroconvulsive Therapy (ECT)
1. Especially for major depression with suicidal ideation that is uncontrolled.

C. Drug therapy
1. Antianxiety and antipanic agents
   a. benzodiazepines
   b. selective serotonin reuptake inhibitors (SSRIs)
2. Antidepressants
3. Antipsychotics (neuroleptics, psychotropic's)
   a. Prolixin
   b. Haldol
4. Hypnotics

5. Mood stabilizers (lithium)
6. Stimulants

V. Closing Statement:

The primary mental illnesses that exist within our society, ones that cause the most disturbing byproduct, are largely the ones regarding psychotic behavior; namely, schizophrenia & bipolar illnesses. While the others are also important, it would be a great relief if we could find the cause for schizophrenia. Probably a better word would be schizophrenias. The plurality of the word reveals to us that the disease is not just one syndrome, but many. Perhaps finding just that one would also reveal many others. We can only hope.

Although the book "The Language of Medicine, Chabner" is an excellent one, I have written a book with the title, "Medical Terminology by the Mnemonic Story System," that can be used as a supplement for the long course or as a primary text for distant learning. An example of chapter two follows.

CHAPTER TWO—MNEMONICS

ELEMENT *MEANING*	MNEMONIC DEVICE	ASSOCIATION-IMAGE
ab-(ab)	able	Although an *able* combat veteran Joe could not get far enough *away from* spiders. It was a real phobia.	*away from, not.*

This prefix takes the form a—before m, p, and v, and abs—before c and t.

Examples: abnormal—away from normal; departing from normal.

abneural—passing away from a nerve (usually to a muscle).

avulsion—"a pulling away from," as in an avulsion fracture.

abscond—to run away from, esp. to freedom.

| acoust(i)- (a-coost-ee) | A costly | I *hear* that the movie with the new *sound* is a costly production. | *hearing, sound.* |

Because of the familiarity of acousti—in words, this form has been chosen to present the root. However, the basic root meaning sound is acous—or acus-.

Example: -acusis—used to denote a condition of hearing (also—*acusia*).

| acro-
(ak-row) | acronym | Imagine the acronym SCUBA with extremities swimming under water. | *extremities; tip;end a top or peak.* |

Note that whatever the reference, "extremity" or acro—always includes the farthest ends and all parts leading to the farthest ends.

| aden-
(a-den) | laden | Certain parts of our body are laden with glands that function to fulfill a specific function. | *gland (e.g. urine).* |

	Examples:	adenic—pertaining to a gland or the glands.
		adenopathy—any disease of a gland.
		adenosis—any condition of a gland.

| adnexa-
(ad-neks-ah) | add next | You may add next the following: two ties connected with a red bow. | *ties, connections, appendage or adjacent parts.* |

This word is a combination of the prefix ad—meaning "to" plus the root nex—meaning "join." Literally, the word means "joined to" and is applied chiefly to refer to the ocular adnexa, the appendages to the eye such as the lacrimal apparatus, and the uterine adnexa, the appendages or adjacent parts of the womb such as the ovaries, the uterine tubes and ligaments.

| | Examples: | adnexopexy (adnex/o/pexy)—the operation of fixing the uterine adnexa to the abdominal wall. |

adnexitis (adnex/itis)—inflammation of the uterine adnexa.

| aer-
(ay-er) | are | He said, "You are nothing but a windbag, Sir, full of hot air." | *air* |

| | Examples: | Aerial—pertaining to air
aeropathy (aer/o/pathy)—"bends"
aerosis (aer/o/sis)—production of gas in the tissues or organs. | |

| -algia
(al-jee-ah) | Al, gee | Oh Al, gee, I wish you no pain, but you're on my foot. | *pain, painful condition* |

The element-algia may be further separated into two parts: Literally (-ia) "condition of" and (alg-) "pain,"—*algia* is the most frequent form expressing pain. However, *alg*—is a root meaning "pain" and can appear in other forms such as algesi-, algo-, algeo- algio-.

| | Examples: | algospasm (alg/o/spasm)—painful, involuntary contraction; painful cramp.
algiomuscular (algi/o/muscular)—causing painful muscular movements.
myalgia (my/algia)—pain in muscle. | |

| alveol-
(al-vee-ol) | Al & Viola | Al & Viola are having a sock-it to me contest to see who can hit the other in the solar plexus cavity. | *cavity, socket small cavity, pit or hollow.* |

This root is used most frequently to refer to the cavities or sockets of either jaw in which the roots of the teeth are embedded.

Examples: alveolus (alveol/us)—(plural alveoli) name used to designate a small saclike pit or cavity; dental alveoli—the tooth sockets in the upper and lower jaw bones.

alveolar (alveol/ar)—pertaining to an alveolus.

ambi-
ambo-
(am-bee-oh)

Bambi

Bambi seemed trapped. *both, on both* There was bamboo *sides around* fence on both sides, but he could jump the smallest one to safety.

You may know that ambi/dextrous means equal ease in using both hands. Compare with the concept extrovert and introvert. What would an ambivert be?

Examples: ambi/sexual—pertaining to or affecting both sexes

ambi/ent—surrounding, on both or all sides.

ameb-
(ah-me'bah)

ameba

When looking through *change* a microscope you can see the one-cell'ed ameba change shape as it moves.

Examples: ameba, amoeba (ameb/a, amoeb/a)—a one-celled animal which moves by constantly changing its shape amebic (ameb/ic)—pertaining to, or of the nature of, an ameba.

amebiasis (ameb/ia/sis)—infestation with amebas, especially intestine.

| amphi- ampho-(am'fe) | Am free | Some say I am free because I can move around on both sides of my internal world of mind; left and right, as if in two ways of thinking. | *both, in two ways, roundabout, Around.* |

An amphi/theater is an oval U-shaped structure surrounded by rows of seats.

An amphi/bi/an can live in two environments.

| | Examples: | amphi/cran/ia—pain on both sides of the head (Taber's) amph/o/dipl/op/ia—double vision in both eye. | |

| an-, a-(an) | an a | John brought home a report card without an A, not one A. Was he lacking in some way? | *without, not/ lacking; weakness; deficiency.* |

| | Note: | The form of the prefix is an—before vowels (a, e, i, o, u and usually h); the form is a—before the consonants. | |

| | Examples: | anemia (an/em/ia)—"lack of blood"; lack of red cells in the blood. anesthesia (an/esthesia)—"lack of feeling"; unconsciousness. avitaminosis (a/vitamin/osis)—"lack of vitamins"; vitamin deficiency. | |

Communication and Living

atrophy (a/trophy)—"lacking development, growth"; a wasting away.

(an'je)	angi-Angie	When Angie does her daily exercise the blood vessels in her legs stand out like mini road maps.	*vessel, usually, blood.*
	Note:	While the principal reference is to blood vessels, angi—can also designate tubes, ducts, or canals which convey the fluids of the body.	
	Examples:	angiitis (angi/itis)—inflammation of a vessel, usually blood.	
		angiomegaly (angi/o/megal/y)— enlargement of the vessels.	
		angiosis (angi/osis)—any condition of the vessels.	
ante- (an'tee)	ante up	In the card game of poker you usually ante up with your bet before the cards are dealt.	*before, in time; or in space.*
	Note:	This prefix appears in a much—used form of anter/o—which is restricted to the meaning "before in space" or "forward" usually meaning *direction.*	
	Examples:	antepartum (ante/part/um)— occurring before birth.	
		anterior (anter/ior)—situated more toward the front, belly surface.	

anteroposterior (anter/o/poster/ior)—from front to back as in AP & Lat film of the chest.

anti- (an'tie)	auntie	I hear that your Auntie Elsie is against abortion.	*against, opposing, (acting against).*

Examples: antigen (anti/gen)—a substance that, when introduced into the body, stimulates the "production of" an "opposing" substance called an anti/body.

antalgesic (ant-al-je'-sik)—pain-relieving agent.

antacid (ant/acid)—a substance that counteracts acidity.

antr- (an'ter)	enter	Said the spider to the fly, "Enter my chamber and we shall see what cavity have thee!"	*cavity or chamber.*

Examples: antrum (antr/um)—a sinus; a cavity or chamber, especially bone.

antrodynia (antr/o/dyn/ia)—pain in an antrum.

arthr- (ar'thro)	Arthur	King Arthur exclaimed, "It's water on my knee; I doubt I have any beer in the joint!"	*joint, articulation.*

Examples: arthral (arthr/al)—pertaining to a joint

arthroplasty (arthr/o/plast/y)—plastic repair (surgery) of a joint

arthrodesis (arthr/o/desis)—the
surgical fixation of a joint

-asthenia	as the knee	It is a well known fact	*weakness*
(as-the' ne-ah)		that disuse produces	
		atrophy, and, in the	
		leg, it can be seen as	
		the knee that is the	
		smallest is the one with	
		the weakness, the one	
		shrunk from disuse.	

Note: This suffix combination is formed
from three useful elements, the prefix
a—meaning "not" or "lacking"; plus
the root sthen—meaning "strength"
or "strong"; plus the word ending—
ia meaning "morbid (diseased)
condition." Literally, the word can be
translated as "a condition of lacking
strength" or "weakness."

Examples: adenasthenia (aden/asthen/ia)—a
weakness in glandular secretion;
deficient glandular activity.

asthenia (asthen/ia)—lack or loss of
strength, energy.

asthenopia (asthen/op/ia)—a
condition of weakness in the eye.

astr-	astronomy	Astronomy is the study	*star shaped*
(as'tro)		of the heavenly bodies,	
		some of which are star	
		shaped.	

Examples: astrocyte (astr/o/cyt/e)—a star shaped
cell, esp. nervous.

astroid (astr/oid)—star shaped.

aur- (aw'ral)	aura	Jody said, "I can only see her bright blue aura around her left ear."	*ear*
	Examples:	auricle (aur/i/cle)—the projecting part of the ear. auris (aur/is)—the ear.	
auto- (aw-toh)	ought to	Gloria said, "He ought to take care of his self, 'cause no one else will."	*self, self-caused.*
	Examples:	autogenic (auto/gen/ic)—self-producing. autopathy (auto/pathy)—a disease without external cause. autoplasty (auto/plasty)—grafting from patient's own body.	
benign (be-nine)	be mine	Be mine, *mild* or hot, for only love, not love me not, can serve us both.	*mild, not cancerous.*
	Note:	The principal use of the word is to designate the absence of cancerous tumors as in "a benign tumor" versus "a carcin/oma."	
bili- (bill-eh)	Billy	Billy had a plan most vile, without a smile, the gall of him!	*bile*
	Examples:	biliary (bili/ary)—pertaining to bile or collectively to the bile, bile ducts, and gallbladder	

biliuria (bili/uria)—bile in the urine

blephar- (blef-ar)	bluffer	One can often tell a poker bluffer by the twitch in his eyelids.	*eyelids*
	Examples:	blepharospasm (blephar/o/spasm)—involuntary movements (contractions) of the eyelid. blepharitis (blephar/itis)—inflammation of an eyelid.	
brachy- (brack-ee)	break	The class took a short break before starting again.	*short*
	Examples:	brachy/meta—measurably short. brachy/faci/al—low, broad face. brachy/gnath/ia—abnormal shortness of the under jaw.	
brady- (brad-ee)	Brady	Imagine watching one hour of the TV show The Brady Bunch in slow motion; almost hypnotic.	*slow*
	Examples:	bradycardia (brady/card/ia)—abnormal slowness of the heartbeat (usually < 60 beats per minute). bradyglossia (brady/glossia)—abnormal slowness of utterance. bradylogia (brady/log/ia)—abnormal slowness of speech due to slowness of thinking, as in a mental disorder.	

bucc(o)- (buk-ko)	buck	A burr under the saddle will very likely cause a horse to buck with nostrils flared and cheeks puffed as you fall on your nether cheeks; oh, the pain!	*cheek*
	Examples:	buccal (bucc/al)—pertaining to the cheek. bucally (bucc/al/ly)—toward the cheek.	
burso- (bur-so)	burro	Jacob put the pack sack on the burro with care, as Jenny the burro was skittish.	*sac (usually* *with a* *lubricating* *fluid).*
	Examples:	bursitis (burs/itis)—inflammation of a bursa. bursopathy (burso/path/y)—any disease of the bursa.	
calc- (cal-sik)	caulk	He filled the seam with caulk using the heel of his hand to press it firmly into the stone crevice.	*heel, stone*
	Examples:	calcemia (calc/emia)—excess of calcium in the blood. calcic (cal/cic)—pertaining to calcium or lime.	

| cantho-
(kan-tho) | can though | The angle at the end of my eyelid is not for me to see, but you can, though. | *angle at the end of the eyelid <o>.* |

Examples: canthal (canth/al)—pertaining to a corner of the eye.

canthus (canth/us)—name of the corner of the eye.

CHAPTER TWO—ELEMENT APPERCEPTION EXERCISE

Pronounce the word aloud, and then break down the word into its elements. Define the elements by stating the meaning of the last element first, then the others in order.

Example: Word = Auto/brady/asthen/ia = weakness, slow, self or a slow weakness of self. This word does not exist. Do you think that it could, or will in the future?

1. abneural	20. avulsion
2. blepharalgia	21. acoustics
3. acroadenalgia	22. aerasthenia[29]
4. alveolalgia	23. adenopathy
5. adenosis	24. adnexopexy
6. algospasm	25. algiomuscular
7. alveolus	26. ambisexual
8. amebic	27. amebiasis
9. amphicrania	28. amphodiplopia
10. anesthesia	29. bursoalgia (dynia)[30]
11. angiomegaly	30. antepartum

---

[29] Also Psychasthenia: Loss of self confidence and mental worry seen in pilots.
[30] Dynia to be covered in later lesson. It also means pain.
[31] Osis refers to "condition of", and is in Lesson Eight.

12. anteroposterior

13. antigen

14. arthrodesis

15. asthenopia

16. autogenic

17. brachygnathia

18. bursopathy

19. canthal

31. abarthrosis[31]

32. antrodynia

33. adenasthenia

34. antibrachium

35. biliuria

36. bradylogia

37. calcemia

38. cantholysis

Meaning Point:

Many medical words by direct definition do not carry a meaning identical with the roots or elements therein contained. When a word, such as psychasthenia does not seem to make sense, look it up.

As the name of the book implies, there must also be stories included that assist with remembering. At the end of some of the chapters, the student is given the chance to find medical words imbedded within a story. An example follows.

PRACTICAL EXERCISE IN THE STORY TEST

This is an exercise that you can do to practice your skill at deciphering (in story format), the medical terms taken from the first three chapters. In this test, you will find a short story-vignette made up of the association/images found in the first three lessons. There are eight (8) word elements to be found (usually you will have 10). Not all paragraphs will contain an association/image that refers to a medical word element. At the end of the story, put down in the appropriate paragraph number the medical word element that you believe is indicated. Remember, the words that you put down are medical word elements, not lay terms. There is no answer sheet in this book. Before you have your first 100-element test this exercise will be covered in class. Again, if you have any questions, please bring them up in class.

BEAUTY AND THE ACE

1. There is a story told of a young woman by the name of Geraldine who needed money to pay off her mortgage. Somehow, she had gotten herself into a poker game with four men. We pick up the story after several hands of straight 5-card draw poker. Nothing is wild, except, perhaps, the fire in Geraldine's red hair.

2. Geraldine looked across the table into McDermat's eyes. One can often tell a poker bluffer by the twitch in his eyelids.

3. McDermat and Geraldine were head-to-head with the highest pot of the evening. All others had folded. The game was five card no draw, no peek; all cards face down, one card up before each bet. Ordinarily, in the card game of poker you ante-up with your bet before the cards are dealt. Then you can raise according to subsequent deals. In no

peek, you put out an "ante", and betting after each card is turned face up.

4. It was McDermat's bet. He had three aces and one queen showing. Geraldine had four kings showing. McDermat was betting that he had an ace down. McDermat pinched each coin to micro-thinness, why, even his skin was thin. Then he threw the coin into the pot. It was a 100-dollar gold piece.

5. McDermat's raise was too high. It was an unfair raise; he wanted her to fold. He was rotten to the core, and that was the heart of the matter.

6. McDermat mumbled to himself, looking at Geraldine across the table, "She is cute, but remember, beauty is only skin deep."

7. Geraldine wrote out an IOU, placed it in the pot and turned over her last card. She delightedly stated, "The card is the ace of hearts!"

8. McDermat pulled a derringer out of his sleeve. A chill shot through the smoke-filled air. Then, he pointed the derringer to his own head and said, "If one puts a gun to his head, and therefore his brain, and pulls the trigger, he could end self and all!" What a poor loser.

9. Someone standing close to McDermat grabbed the derringer away from him, stating, "It isn't any secret, crying over spilled milk is a waste of time."

10. Well, as the story goes, Geraldine paid off her mortgage and McDermat never played another card game again, but instead, became a model citizen. So all is well that ends with the ace of hearts.

It is time to try your skill at completing this exercise by putting down the medical word element indicated in the story for each paragraph below. There are only eight. Allow yourself about 15 minutes. Questions should be brought up in class.

Paragraph Number 1 _____

Paragraph Number 2 _____

Paragraph Number 3 _____

Paragraph Number 4 _____

Paragraph Number 5 _____

Paragraph Number 6 _____

Paragraph Number 7 _____

Paragraph Number 8 _____

Paragraph Number 9 _____

Paragraph Number 10 _____

The appendices of the medical terminology book give special information on how to S.O.A.P.[32] a patient. This relates to the writing of notes, first an example of narrative format for a neuropsychiatric note:

Simple Narrative Communication
As Initial Progress Notes
In a Neuropsychiatric Setting

The first note written should be as complete as time will allow, but as well, there is usually a mandated format. Progress notes must document the presenting problem, the plan for subsequent service, and the indication of some kind of medical necessity. This information may not be required for every progress note, but must reflect new information or changes to information as they occur.

What I shall do in this paper is to give clue to several mnemonic devices that will assist one with remembering. An acceptable narrative format can be developed that will satisfy most audit inquiries.

For just a moment let us look back at the beginning statement, this is a statement of what should be in a note, especially a first note. All primary notes share a commonality of purpose, they tell what happened to whom, when, where, what is to be done by whom, and why this is so; therefore, implicating some kind of necessity/urgency requiring a plan of action. We

---

[32] *Subjective*, patient's own words. *Objective*, exam. *Assessment*, diagnosis. *Plan*, what is to be done.

cannot all be like Capt. Picard of the star ship Enterprise saying with a swish of the finger, "Make it so!" We have to write it down in the record so that someone else will know what we know. More importantly, for someone like an auditor, who knows nothing about the client/patient, other than what he can glean from the record he has before him; therefore, if not written, it did not happen. From skimpy descriptions of poorly organized notes comes the stuff of audit exceptions. I know few auditors that will take the time to look through a record trying to find material to support a note's medical necessity; it is not enough to say, "But Sir it is all there somewhere in the record." This is especially true of that first note. An admission note must be able to stand-alone. This is important whether it be a nursing note, an intake note, or a first note in a nonclinical setting.

In Search of a Style:

To say that we all must write using the same format would be an untruth. Better to say that we should all be putting down the essential information to assist anyone who reads the record in understanding the key factors that brought the patient here at this time, a plan for continuing the treatment and the reason this visit meets medical necessity. The use of a mnemonic device allows one the best use of memory.

One mnemonic device that has been around for a long time is S.O.A.P. (Subjective, Objective, Assessment and Plan). Another was S.P.A.R. (Service, Problem, Action and Result).

One might want to develop guidelines taken directly from the manual, or given protocol where one works, into a useful mnemonic device. Put this information on a 3x5 card and carry it until memorized. As an example, if the manual calls for the following information:

1. Date of service with time in minutes,
2. Service provided,
3. Location of service,
4. Brief narrative, and
5. Description of changes in individual's medical necessity.

The date, time, location and type of service with appropriate numbers, codes, minutes etc. is self-contained in progress record format. However, the narrative description of the patient *event* needs some brief consistency put on paper. It is my firm belief that a single line starting all notes written with that very consistency will exist by using the following mnemonic device: ARSENAL, (Age, race, sex, enters, new or not new, affect and looks, as in facies/attire.

Examples Using Psychiatric Backdrop:

25-y.o. male enters new to system with chief complaint (CC) of suicidal ideation with sad affect and look.

35-y.o. black female enters, not new to the system, with CC of not being able to sleep, affect appropriate to situation, and she looks tired with poor hygiene.

40-y.o. Caucasian female enters, not new to system, with CC of hearing voices with agitated affect and bizarre and unkempt look about her.

80-y.o. Caucasian male enters, not new to system, as danger to others after threatening to kill wife, affect angry with threatening look/actions about self requiring five-point restraint.

15-y.o. Caucasian female enters new to system as danger to self after threatening to take her life with a knife, affect depressed with sad tearful and distraught look.

Obviously, the first line is only a beginning. Now you need to flesh-out the narrative to satisfy the remaining requirements pertaining to the plan for subsequent service or continuing care whether by visit or by bedside or clinic. Another mnemonic device that is often used is:

Hx: History of presenting problem/complaint,
MSE: Mental status exam (for neuropsychiatric),
Dx Imp: Diagnostic impression, and
Plan: What you plan to do by number:

1. Refer to doctor or another service by consult etc.,
2. Give a return visit,
3. Ongoing visits, or
4. Lab or x-ray.

Using an example given for a psychiatric patient in the foregoing, a written example is shown below.

40-y.o. Caucasian female enters, not new to system, (often this may be restated as for a first visit, or repeat visit) with CC of hearing voices with agitated affect and bizarre, unkempt look about herself.

Hx: Client brought by a police officer to outpatient department. It was reported that client had approached this officer stating, "I must inform you that you are in danger. God has sent me to warn you. I just spoke to God and he said that I should tell you that you will die unless you bring me to the mental health clinic." Client has a long history of mental illness and has had a recent admission to a psychiatric health facility within the last two months. Client admitted to not taking her medication because it makes her crazy.

MSE: On examination, client admits to hearing voices, especially of God. She answers questions only after conferring with God. At some level of consciousness she is aware that she needs help; therefore, her reason for approaching the police officer. She is concrete and fearful with a paranoid flavor to her speech. Her primary delusion has to do with her dystonic (bad voices) voices and eventuates in behavior not appropriate in normal social contact. For this reason, she is considered gravely disabled.

Dx Imp: 295.34—Schizophrenia, paranoid, with acute exacerbation, verified by past medical history.

Plan: Detain (5150) for admission to psychiatric health facility.

All that needs to be done at this point is to verify that all the information needed exists; therefore, eluding the knife of audit exception.

Progress notes must document the *presenting problem*, the plan for *subsequent service*, and the reason to believe the patient meets *medical/service necessity*.

1. Presenting problem = CC of hearing voices with agitated affect and bizarre, unkempt look about herself.
2. Plan for subsequent service = Detain for admission to psychiatric service.
3. Reason to believe the patient meets medical/service necessity = on examination client admits to hearing voices, especially God. She is concrete and fearful with a paranoid flavor to her speech. She is delusional with dystonic voices. She may be a danger to self. (Not noted, perhaps implied) She is gravely disabled.

All the essential information exists in the primary note. It stands alone. While the primary note must stand alone, it is not necessary for the following notes to do so. Following information in this chart must reflect new changes in behavior and care. The baseline is drawn. One has only to review the chart to catch a flavor of the beginning and see how the treatment has changed the patient's behavior until time of possible discharge. State laws and mandated performance regarding the determination of medical necessity will be the guidelines of tomorrow. Not every situation is the same. Using mnemonic devices may assist with consistency that will dull the sharp edge of audit exception.

An ambulatory health care philosophy is also included in lesson plan format.

An Introduction to Ambulatory Health Care Philosophy
(Following Information May Require Reader to have some medical training)

Stating a philosophy may predispose one to reveal his or her underlying biases, demonstrate interpretations gathered from many sources found inherently interwoven into the subject; or, in my case, represent many years of gathering information, taking histories, counseling, and working within the disciplines of orthopaedics, neuropsychiatry, and general medicine. Whatever the fundamental disciplines may have been, the philosophical metamorphosis that results must give rise to certain aspects of ambulatory health care that may otherwise go unnoticed, unheeded, or become lost forever leaving those that follow to gain their own foothold without the help of the stepping stones found and used by the many who came before. The nature of humankind is in the unique ability to communicate, to be a time-gathering creature. Gathering together one's thoughts and casting them into the timeless sea of knowledge, hoping that these many fragmented segments of life's experience will somehow take root, grow and replenish humankind with new data to serve, save and preserve.

In support of the foregoing, I shall devote time to three paradigms:

1. The nursing care philosophy and self,

2. Establishing common verbal bonds with the patient, and

3. Taking a history with the patient in mind. (This will include the very specific history and total "s.o.a.p.ing" technique for a low back pain.)

Behavioral Objectives:

1. Briefly discuss or identify the interpersonal or the interaction process with patients as it applies to the following:

    a. Nursing care philosophy and self,
    b. Initial patient interview, obtaining a history, and
    c. Overall screening process, S.O.A.P.ing the patient from start to finish.

2. Briefly describe or identify the procedure used to perform the examination of the patient with the following: Low back pain, Cold, Flu, and specific trauma to the lower and upper extremities to include at a minimum the following:

    a. Taking the history,
    b. Doing the exam,
    c. Deciding on an assessment,
    d. Plan of action including treatment and follow-up care when necessary, and
    e. Final disposition.

Nursing Care Philosophy and Self:

Over the years, I have often asked students to take time from their studies to put together, in 500 words or less, their personal philosophy of life. For many it was a first time for this kind of thought. For some this assignment produced a startling realization that a philosophy per se, did not exist, that life was spent against the cool winds of time. For others, it catalyzed a process already begun. For all, it gave temporary meaning to one of their moments in time, and provided direction for new thought and action, a reference point in their hierarchy of being. Nevertheless, the assignment made, they would bring them to me, the apologetic, the blushing, the dogmatic, the God fearing, the not so God fearing, the early, and the late. I read them all. Some spoke of courage. Many gave clue to a vision of the future, an insight about tomorrow seen today. They spoke of young men and women needing strength to fight their common foes, disease, ignorance, and misunderstanding. Each seemed to be aware of life and the need for love. Finally, much was said about the art of understanding through language and education. They all thought. They all gave something of themselves.

As you might imagine, their words in 500 or less, did not solve all the ills of our world, and they were unable to come up with any magic cures for the common maladies that inflict humankind. Instead, each in their own way, young minds, began a journey into the chilling questions of "why," and for one single moment given a look at "self," and having made this internal journey, they would never again be the same.

A few would leave this place, their inner self-found to be in conflict with the outside reality. Others would go on to finish (in those days a forty week course), while one or two would become truly self-actualized. As instructors, we would come to know a great deal about each one who passed this way. You see, they would leave a great deal of their self-behind. In this process of being here, we would come to know much about their individual philosophies. We, as instructors, would be able to see with some clarity the workings of the inner self as it struggled against the backdrop of nursing. The environment would bring out what was hidden from view. The course would bring out what was unknown. A working agreement with both must develop early if one is to stay in the flow of things. It is at this point that many began to revise their internal philosophies about life and living, and about dying. They are the ones that were able to achieve their end, graduation. What was it that they found out that kept them in the course for forty weeks?

If you expect an answer to the foregoing question that will enable you to achieve graduation without work, dream on. I suspect that students had their individual story to relate. Ones of tears, sweat, and blood, stories that may tell of wrongs and bleached rights, of fare and foul play. Each student would have his say of the instructors. All would have their say about the course. What would make this all worthwhile is the fact that after forty weeks with this school, this faculty, there would be a change in each that would be noticed. Perhaps an inner glow would give its self away. Or, a certain body carriage, but always, deep within there would be a knowledge of self that was not there before; and, a devotion to nursing that would only be seen as time would allow as each graduate traveled the path of life into the future and through the tangled vines of living. Then, each person reflecting on some of what had gone on *here in this place;* and then, each one taking their place in the flow of nursing. Finally, each one becoming only what they could become with such a past, fully actualized, fully alive, and caring for humankind with love in their heart. This concept is better described in the following creed. It is a statement of what I feel many must come to feel if they are to be self actualized, fully involved, a valid part of nursing and life. *At this point, my personal creed is printed, see page 96.*

Establishing Common Verbal Bonds

1. <u>Teaching</u>: Part of what you will be doing is to teach the patient since the medical jargon is not common to the laity. Do this in such a way that you do not insult your patient, or in any way be condescending. Health teaching can be a very rewarding experience.

2. <u>Identifying</u>: You will have to identify the patient's value system in order to relate to him/her. His feedback will give clue to his background, education, and emotional state of the moment. Give him/her his/her say, don't crowd him/her with questions, make value judgments about his/her grammar or way of speaking, interrupt him/her as he/she speaks, that is, allow him/her to finish what he/she is saying. You will understand better, and he/she will feel better. You may identify something very special about each patient if you allow them the freedom of expression without

causing him/her to guard, or in some way to splint his/her thoughts with things he/she feels YOU want to hear. If his/her value system is too foreign or seems incongruous to you, ask for help.

3. Describing: You will be called upon to describe the complaint in terms that can be understood by the patient, however remember, that you do so with the permission of the P.A., or doctor only if you are aware of their philosophy in treating patients. You will have to understand how much each patient needs to know and if allowed to tell it. Be clear on this. For to tell the patient something that he/she cannot handle at the time, may cause irrevocable mental anxiety, or even create an obstinate neurosis. To designate one as a psychosomatic is for the diagnostically destitute. Remember also, that in order to describe you must KNOW and know the actual, not the supposed. Do not tell your patient stories. If you do not know, find out. If you tell a patient that you are going to do a certain thing, then please do it. This is called follow-through.

4. Accepting: You should accept the patient as a person without making moral or value judgments about his/her: station in life, cause of illness, or any shade of difference that may separate him/her from you as you believe yourself to be. If you cannot do this, then you should allow yourself an out, perhaps an out from nursing.

5. Loving: That in its broadest sense, and within the limits of your beliefs or philosophy, you should demonstrate that

you care. Moreover, that you care about what happens, what should be done now, and of the outcome, if it is within your control. Your actions, speech, and demeanor should demonstrate this. For those of you who find it difficult to "pretend," at least make an honest effort to "do." Perhaps in doing you will begin to care, and in caring you will begin to glow with what the patient will feel is genuine concern. If you cannot feign even a modicum of caring, or actually give a damn, then you may like mechanics better.

If the above five steps are incorporated into your clinical acumen they will have a positive effect on you patient-nurse relationship that will go a long way into the process of getting the patient well before any treatment is given. Remember, patients often begin to feel better as soon as they enter into the treatment arena. Why not capitalize on this placebo effect, and create an atmosphere in which this feeling can flourish. Your rewards will be many, and your patient's return visits will be fewer in number and frequency.

Taking a History (Chief Complaint) with the Patient in Mind

1. <u>Do Not Argue</u>: This is no time to argue with patients about their belief, cause of illness, reason of accident, or whatever. You may wish to teach later, or do health teaching now if they have a problem that represents lack of care or knowledge about their body, health, or condition. However, please do not be harsh in your manner or critical in your way of helping. You are not their stern parent figure, but instead, a compassionate human being that has chosen to

be in the health care profession, and by all other standards, no better than they are.

2. <u>Own Words</u>: When taking a history from a patient, use his/her own words with any necessary clarification of word meaning or choice. Use quotation marks to set off their thoughts, descriptions, and phrases.

3. <u>Use Format</u>: If possible, follow some kind of format or outline until you learn the necessary steps and questions using mnemonic devices, forms, especially the ones within this article on low back pain, they will save you time and assist with an assessment.

4. <u>Be Attentive</u>: Listen to your patient. Do not be so rude as to write, without making eye contact, talk to someone else, or discuss another patient on your present patient's time. If you find it difficult to remember what a patient tells you, take short notes on a separate pad and then transfer these to the form later, or during a pause. This means that you must maintain eye contact with your patient as much as is possible. If you are interrupted by a peer, ask if urgent, if not, tell him/her that you will be available as soon as you are through. Give your patient his/her due time. However, remember, there will be times when a patient will want more than his/her share of your time. It will be your job to find a way to terminate the interview without making the patient feel slighted or cheated. When you can put out your hand to a patient, and they take it, then you will know that you have earned yourself a place in the treating

environment worth keeping. Nevertheless, when a patient tells you "thank you" as well, you have reached a threshold in your clinical acumen that you can call self actualized, at least for the moment. There are many moments in the day of a nurse.

5. <u>Taber's Cyclopedic Medical Dictionary</u> has an interpreter index in five languages that may aid you in asking questions for those who do not speak English well; but also, this book will help you with the various meanings of many medical words.

Low Back Pain as an Isolated Entity
Written in lesson plan format

I. Introduction:
   A. <u>Opening Statement</u>: When man chose to stand erect, to stand on his hind legs and work against the ever-constant pull of gravity with his quadrupedal motor skeletal equipment, man fell heir to the frequent inadequacies of that equipment, presupposing him to low back pain. While it is true that he has gained two hands, it is also true that he has now only two feet to do the work of four. The penalty will forever reside within the confines of his aching lower back. Let us look into some of the consequences of poor body mechanics, selective overloading, and the much talked about trauma of everyday living.

B. Objectives:

1. Identify and/or briefly describe three causes of chronic low back pain.

2. Briefly describe and/or identify the procedure used for the taking of a history (chief complaint), performing the examination, the making of an assessment (provisional diagnosis), and the plan of action for a patient with the chief complaint of low back pain.

C. Procedure and Lesson tie-in (if used for class presentation): This instruction is given in preparation for the following hours on physical assessment and examination during the screening process. The steps in the low back exam will be done and will be used as an example to demonstrate the entire procedure of taking a history (chief complaint), doing an exam, forming an impression (assessment and/or diagnosis), and discerning a valid treatment, or deciding to refer the patient to a specialist for final disposition.

II. Explanation:
   A. Causes of low back pain (chronic and acute)[33]

   1. Low back pain of postural origin:
      a. Poor body mechanics may account for the largest portion seen.

---

[33] *Trauma,* McLauglin, W.B. Saunders & Co., 1960, Chapter 21.

b. Selective overloading of the anti gravity skeletal muscle system is the strain you can produce by over working one muscle group, especially using a cold muscle or one group because of poor mechanical advantage.

c. Poor muscle tone or disuse atrophy. As in, because of improper use or disuse of the vastus medialis, injury to the knee occurs, as it is difficult to fully extend the leg to its only stable position.

d. Overweight.

2. Myositis and Fibrositis:

a. An inflammation caused from disease or old or recent trauma.

b. This process exists within muscle and connective tissue. It may be superficial or deep causing pain at a distance from the origin. Many times pinching massage will bring it out.

3. Osteoarthritis:

a. If called a disease, occurs usually after forty years of age. Pain may be caused by an unknown factor, or be the result of past trauma, whether a gradual insult over time, or a sudden one within a few hours.

b. It is a process of the normal aging of the adult.

c. Usually centers its pain producing problems within the joints of the extremities. When this is so, it will be called by a special name. Reference: Arthritis, Tenosynovitis. Etc.

4. Unstable Lumbosacral Spine:
   a. Congenital defects.
   b. Transitional presacral vertebra (L-5, S-1). Common anomaly exhibits structural characteristics of both a last lumbar and a first sacral segment. It can be fused or have a joint interposed between the transverse process of the presacral vertebra and sacrum.
   c. Disc disease and/or trauma, as in HNP.

B. Taking a history for low back pain complaint (example): (Notes written verbatim)

1. Sample History: 25 y/o cau male with hx of low back pain last 24 hours, stating that he has had no injury within the last five years. Patient remembers helping to lift heavy tent the day before the episode. However, he denies pain at the time of lifting. Pain began the following morning after getting out of bed. Pain made worse by standing and lifting things. Pain seems to respond to heat and being flat on back. Patient's daily habits and job: works at a desk all day, does very little exercise during the week. Plays some handball and used to lift weights. Pain is located low back and does not radiate into either leg. Patient was seen for a similar type pain over five years ago. He was not

hospitalized. He does not remember if he was given any medication at that time. Was told to exercise, but does not remember how. He is not taking any medication at present. Patient appears to be in good health and walks with a list to the left. Patient is 6'0" weighing 200 pounds. No other complaints described. Any family history of bone disease may well fit in at this point. Be sure to watch the patient's affect, posture, and listen to the words that he uses to describe his malady.

C. Physical Exam (objective data) patient with CC low back pain:

1. Use chronological record of care form.
2. Guide to Physical Exam

a. Spine Alignment: Objective signs of LBP are loss of normal lumbar loridosis called flattening, or a lateral list causing asymmetry of the lorodotic line.

b. Muscle Spasm defining the erector spinae muscles palpable as prominent hard cord in a position of maximum stretch. Some may say that there is no spasm in the back. Describe what you feel and can see.

c. Mobility of trunk: (ROM) Loss of motion in the quadrupedal position, usually in the lorodotic region. Loss of ROM in flexion and/or extension with some associated pelvic tilt. Using a plumb bob one may calculate how much pelvic tilt or shortening of the lower extremity exists.

d. <u>Deep Tendon Reflexes</u> (DTRs): Biceps, C-5 level; Triceps, C-6 level; Radial, C-8 level; Ulnar, T-1 level; Patellar, L-2 & 3 level; and the achilles, L-5—S1 level.

e. <u>ROM Exercises</u>: SLR, straight leg raising; WLR, weight load resistance; Sit-ups with legs straight and also with hip flexed; Heel-toe walking to test for strength of the muscles supplied by the nerves mentioned in (d), and to define any existing paresis or imbalance.

f. <u>Sensation</u>: "Normal" feeling within each lower extremity. This is a subjective data since you will have to ask the patient.

g. <u>Atrophy</u>: Check one muscle group against the opposite side, usually the thigh group or the calf group is chosen. Measure an equal distance from a known body landmark, mark with pen, and use a tape measure to determine the girth of the muscle mass. Palpation of some muscles during use may give clue as well.

h. <u>Sciatic Pain</u>: Attachment of the hamstring muscles to the pelvis flexes the lumbosacral joint and stretches the paravertebral soft tissue putting tension on the sciatic nerve. Certain motions of the hamstring muscles will bring out pain in a tender inflamed sciatic nerve. If the nerve has been traumatized, it will also be tender. Direct pressure with a blunt instrument or digit may bring pain along the sciatic distribution as well. During straight leg raising, dorsiflexion of the foot may bring out sciatic pain, and if so, this should be noted. Sciatic pain, whatever the method used to elicit, must be evaluated.

D. Forming an Impression (Dx or Assessment):

1. After taking an accurate history and doing a rather complete exam, which should take about 15 minutes, an assessment, or provisional diagnosis, will naturally follow. Some low back complaints will take longer than 15 minutes. If there has been a history of recent injury or the patient has been seen by someone the day before you will have to make some changes in your format. If the patient is in pain from an injury, you may want to defer part of your exam. In the absence of obvious disability, a referral to a specialist may be indicated. At that point, it is necessary not to create further trauma.

2. The assessment is based on ruling out specific entities, especially neurological and/or traumatic findings. In the presence of any positive findings, a specialist or doctor should make the final disposition.

3. The following assessments made most often:
   a. Lumbosacral strain,
   b. Lumbosacral strain with muscle spasm,
   c. Lumbosacral pain, etiology unknown,
   d. Low back pain of postural origin,
   e. Low back pain (chronic or acute) post traumatic, and
   f. To rule out disc disease.

E. Treating the Isolated Entity:
   1. In the absence of any positive neurological signs, and with a negative history for trauma, treatment will be primarily symptomatic with concern directed to obviate the cause, reeducation of the involved muscles, rest, exercises, and the medication of choice.

   2. Isolation of the offending muscle group may be possible in some cases. When this feat is accomplished, the treatment may be exacting. The treatments listed below are by no means the only ones, for even as I put these words on paper, new ones are being tried somewhere.

      a. Ice massage alone, or on an intermittent basis with heat,
      b. Rest on a firm, thin, mattress, supine or laterally recumbent, not on abdomen,
      c. Pelvic traction,
      d. William's exercises,
      e. Pain medication with muscle relaxant, non-narcotic,

      f. Dichlorotetrafluroethane or ethyl chloride topographically, or Surface anesthesia, similar to ice massages technique,

      g. Injection of a trigger-point with xylocaine and depo-medrol or some other kind of anti-inflammatory medication, and

      h. Patient teaching.

III. Summary:

    A. Review of Main Points:

        1. Causes of low back pain,

        2. Taking a history for low back pain as a chief complaint,

        3. bjective exam,

        4. Forming an assessment, and

        5. Treating the isolated entity.

    B. Closing Statement:

When low back pain is the chief offending complaint, certain observations will point the way to probable cause, and possible treatment. Knowing the possible causes, using a thorough history, and doing the exam should create an environment for positive treatment in all but the most resistant cases. A specialist or an orthopaedic doctor sees lower back syndromes existing outside these confines. A specialist in neurology or orthopaedics will inevitably make final judgment in all equivocal cases. Your job is to see that this determination is made before the offending lesion produces irreversible damage to the patient.

In this paper, I have given clue to the complexities within the treating arena that exist as soon as the patient enters the room. Your job is made complex in no small way because you can speak, think, and form pre judgments in more than just the area concerned with your patient's signs and symptoms; but, equally because you are human and subject to the same feelings, wants, and fears as your patient. Objectivity, though often sought by many clinicians, may not be the answer. Many a machine can give an impression. Emotional involvement does not mean that the loss of effectiveness must follow. Too much of our world today is given to the superficial, "I do not want to become involved," type of verbal, and body communication. We have become cold diagnostic computers aloof, alas, even oblivious to our human surroundings. If one seeks no one, no one need respond. Each patient is part of your life whether you want him or her to be or not. Treat that person as an end in his or her self, for everyone has some value of merit. We are all part of a whole. If you take from that whole, you take from yourself. The reality of living is that we are born needing someone and we will certainly die quite alone without someone to care. Many will come to a clinic for no other reason than needing someone to care, even if for only that moment. The fruits of healing are deeply interwoven with the care given to the mind as well as the body, and the body and soul are one.

Additionally, there is an example of a transcription for an intake shown below.

EXAMPLE OF TRANSCRIPTION
Neuropsychiatric Intake

The following example is not taken from an actual recording, and the information does not relate to any real case history. The information is purely fictional. The subject matter is based on multiple real histories in many manuals, books, and information derived from the DSM-IV (Diagnostic and Statistical Manual of Mental Disorders, 4th Edition), to name only a few. The pathology demonstrated could be real. The situation depicted is fictional. However, as it exists, it gives a realistic representation of the pathology that could exist in such a case history.

IDENTIFYING DATA:

This is my initial contact with this 32-year-old Caucasian female. She is approximately 5'5", buxom, blond, with a pallid complexion. She is dressed in appropriate attire for her age. She is admitted on a 5150 status for psychiatric observation due to an aberrant behavior pattern for the last seven days as well as possible danger to her infant son.

HISTORY OF PRESENT PROBLEM:

The patient came to the attention of her family because "she seemed to be different," according to her husband. After recently (about six weeks) giving birth to a nine-pound-five ounce boy, she began to say strange things and seemed depressed. Primary reason for this first admission has to do with the patient leaving her six-week-old infant alone in his crib and the patient being found in town in a bar trying to engage a male in a sexual liaison. Her reason, she stated, "God has made me the mother of all men. They are just little boys, you know!"

She has no previous mental health history and she is in good physical condition. Childbirth was normal. There are no known problems of childhood and she takes no drugs or alcohol, other than medications prescribed by her family doctor. In fact, her being in the bar was quite unusual, according to her family, as she has never had a drinking problem or ever taken a drink, even on special occasions. She was referred to, by other family members, as being a teetotaler.

MENTAL STATUS EXAM:

The patient presents as petite, immaculate in dress, with a strong odor of perfume and appropriate makeup. She comes to the interview willingly. She offers no complaint, but states, "I'm on a mission to save all men from their sexual fantasies." She offers no reason, other than the one given initially, for her behavior—in fact, does not seem to be aware of the implications of what she has done, stating only that God has spoken to her. She denies suicidal thoughts and is without concomitant suicidal ideation. At times, there is a flight of ideas, and she attends to internal stimuli. She is oriented in time, person, and place. There is grandiosity to her speech content that almost seems bipolar. There is no evidence of memory impairment, confusion, clouding of sensorium, or other signs of organic brain disease or schizophrenia.

DIAGNOSTIC IMPRESSION:

Axis I   298.90 Psychotic Disorder, NOS
          R/O Post Partum Psychosis
          R/O Bipolar Psychosis
Axis II   V71.09 none noted
Axis III Post Partum X six weeks
Axis IV   Stressors 3—moderate (childbirth)
Axis V   Current: 25
          Highest: 80

TREATMENT PLAN:

1. Evaluation for medication after routine tests,
2. The patient will be involved in the general ward milieu,
3. The patient will be involved in individual and group psychotherapy while on the ward, and
4. There should be close collaboration with the patient's family prior to release and an investigation and/or follow-up past history in more detail by social worker while patient is on the ward.

EPILOG

PUTTING IT ALL TOGETHER

After over 35 years of teaching, counseling, and working within the nursing environment, I have developed a theoretical approach to personality development. This would be a good time to put everything together. I will have to take from the earlier chapters, and then embellish the material with cogent review.

My primary emphasis has to do with the statement, what I do. Simplistic, though to the point, an applicable starting point in the destination for defining self from the point of view: what I do is what I am. For men this becomes an ominous truth. Take away what I do reduces one to a kind of nonexistence. This is not a good place to be.

A good starting point is the three pillars of life.

THREE PILLARS OF LIFE

Spirit	**Organic**	**Knowledge**
Religion	*Body*	*Mind*
God	*Flesh*	*Psyche*
Soul	*Chemical*	*Logos*
Weightless	*Carbon*	*Reason*
Eternal	*Finite*	*Tentative*
psychospiritual	**psychochemical**	**psychointellectual**

Assuming that the forgoing is true, in at least some small way, we can venture a guess at some of the combinations that exist within a given personality. Remember, we are talking about men. I do not have a long enough life to include that complex persona that includes women.

The ideal relationship between the three pillars would be 1/3, 1/3, 1/3. This would mean that each would have the same weight. This is much like a statistical average; it probably does not exist per se. The next step would be to hypothesize what some possible relationships would be.

I suppose that I can use myself as an example, I know myself best. First, I must develop a list of traits that make up general personality existence. This will be difficult. Should I select arbitrary traits, ones taken from other personality theories, or make up my own. Let the research begin.

Big Five Personality Traits (Goldberg, 1993)

The Big Five are a descriptive model of personality, not a theory, although psychologists have developed theories to account for the Big Five. Traits have been developed by observations made in language, especially since differences in people's lives will eventually become encoded into their language.

Openness to Experience—appreciation for art, emotion, adventure, unusual ideas, imagination, and curiosity.

Conscientiousness—a tendency to show self-discipline, act dutifully, and aim for achievement; planned rather than spontaneous behavior.

Extraversion—energy, positive emotions, surgency,[34] and the tendency to seek stimulation and the company of others.

Agreeableness—a tendency to be compassionate and cooperative rather than suspicious and antagonistic towards others.

Neuroticism—a tendency to experience unpleasant emotions easily, such as anger, anxiety, depression, or vulnerability; sometimes-called emotional instability.

Reducing personality traits to five is a constriction that might work with the three pillars; at least, it is fewer qualities to juggle. Each one placed against the attributes shown within a pillar.

Psychospiritual—looking at the Big Five I find little reference to God, spirit, soul, et cetera. I have chosen a few words to reference spirit as a quality or belief one has, especially in reference to a supreme being. The closest reference may have to do with *openness to experience*, for in the appreciation for art, emotion et al, there may be a place for the appreciation that we come from somewhere, in that somewhere exists an eternalness, and this thought of the vastness of the universe leads one to the obvious, we are not alone.

It may well be how each one of us encompasses our finiteness, which makes God self-evident, even to the most doubting. Without a single strand of spirit, the soul is denied.

---

[34] **Surgency**—includes leadership and extroversion traits. People strong in surgency like to lead and want to be in charge.

A lacking in this part of the persona creates a cold, distant and calculating person that may act in a Machiavellian way. It can be said that the spirit binds two in love. It makes one wonder why the divorce rate may be as high as 50% in some states, perhaps higher.

Psychochemical—unfortunately, the closest one is *neuroticism*. Energy put into anger, anxiety certainly implicates neurochemical activity. I hate to think that the only relationship has to do with emotional instability as it reeks of mental illness. While this can be the case, the psychochemical component is more the holding place and not the cause. Schizophrenia has a relationship with organicity, as in an organic brain disease. I would not want to think that this is the only reference to the psychochemical part of the triad.

Within the *openness to experience* trait a reference to emotion, imagination, and curiosity may hint at an awareness of the chemical part of self. A thinking that emotion can spring from deep within gives clue to this propensity. *Behavior is caused*. This goes back to the hierarchy of learning:

Change in behavior is the capital fragment of the hierarchy. After wading through years of growth substrata, we come to the process of encoding our language in the light of the present, tinted by past memories and expressed with hope for the future. Above all, our behavior is *caused*. We do not act in a vacuum.

The psychochemical relationship to organic reality may be three-fold, chemical as in pheromone, chemical as in the neurochemistry of the synaptic junction, and at the most fundamental level a neuro-electrical polarity of the cell and DNA. The behavior secondary to psychochemical activation is predictable. When fear activates an adrenalin rush, behavior becomes fight or flight at the most rudimentary level. In the cyclic testosterone balance in men, when high, produces aggressive behavior, when low, the opposite. This part of the triad is necessary to procreation, marriage, and the ability for some to create works of art et cetera.

In short, psychochemical relates to physiological need, the psychointellectual connotes awareness of that need, and psycho spiritual purifies the need by moral reflection. In all, the valence of sexuality is determined by the interacting parts of the personality. When imbalance occurs, or part of the triad is missing there is an aberration in the personality that may lead to a psychological diagnosis.

Psychointellectual—*openness to experience,* where knowledge rules, and in a way from a Freudian point of view may represent the ego. Knowledge is certainly tentative. Psycheintellectual would be a better term, as initially the term psyche related to soul, mind, or spirit. It is then a meld between mind and knowledge. An empty brain is as a vacuum and as such cannot exist in nature. Knowledge of our world is in a constant state of flux, yet we shall never know all.

This part of the personality concerns the learning in three domains. The affective domain—the learning of values and attitudes that can influence beliefs; the cognitive domain—the learning of ideas and factual information; and, the psychomotor domain—the learning of physical skills. These skills become the dominating factor within the three. Knowledge of the world, your worldview and your ability to use that knowledge to benefit self becomes you. However, each part of the triad is weighted, preponderance in any one will show itself as time allows. Your position in organic reality will be shown as you display your dominance in one of the three.

Earlier stated, a 1/3, 1/3, 1/3 relationship would be ideal. I also suggested that I could use myself as an example. Unlike Freud, I will not pretend that my theory represents a scientific fact; rather that it is an introspective delving at best. My search for knowledge has been my life. If that is not evident in my writing, then I have failed miserably.

In evidence is my search for knowledge, and that is factual. In the subterranean matter that is my mind, I have gathered knowledge. Others that know me, and there are few, indicate than I live in a metal world rather than an emotional one. At times, this can be an impediment to my ability to care. It leaves me drenched with the scent of aloneness. This is not always good. If I were to quantify my depth into each of the parts of the triad, it would look like this:

Psychochemical-30%, psychespiritual-20%, and psychointellectual-50%. There are times when the relationships change with a preponderance in the intellectual realm. When I was twenty, the psychochemical part of the triad was probably 60%. With maturation comes change. With change comes maturation. As

I approach ninety, the pillar dominance will change, until there will be a predominance in the psychointellectual I am most sure i.e., if dementia does not intrude.

To determine your level in any of the three make a pie and divide it into three areas. Write in each area a factor that represents, for you, one of each of the three parts of the personality. Now factor in the importance of each to you, for example, love, God, work. For men there is usually a divided loyalty between their work and the love for a woman. Later in life, your work identifies who you are. Without your work, you may cease to exist in the psychological sense. You have become what you do. Suicide in men is more frequent with the absence of a work identity. It follows the pattern of Idealism, Frustration, and Demoralization.[35] A work identity is highly idealized, when gone, frustration and then demoralization. Since taught at an early age that man is what he does, a work-void cannot exist, we may then remove our self from the equation. There are many ways to lose one's work identity. Remember the case of John.

The Case of John

John Doe was a God-fearing man, often times to the extreme. He believed profusely in the golden rule, do unto to others as you would have them do unto you, but do it first. He proclaimed of the Lord Almighty aloud in the midst of others often, and he went to church almost every Sunday. However,

---

[35] *People in Quandaries,* Johnson, Wendell, Harper & Brothers, 1946, pages 14, 18, and 488.

he had issue with the fact that not everyone believed as he did. He would spend time in conversation trying to convince others, especially his close friends. This would often lead to long periods when he would not hear from anyone, not even his close friends. Eventually, he became somewhat of a recluse. One Sunday while attending church service, he noted that the sermon did not agree with some of his underlying principles. He stood abruptly and gave argument, openly and loudly. This eventuated in John leaving the church in a huff. He was no longer welcome in the congregation. More a recluse than ever, he developed agoraphobia and finally was deeply in need of professional help.

This is only part of the equation. What is needed to flesh out the forgoing has to do with John's work identity. If John's job had to do with the church, it is evident; but what if his job was teaching in a community college. A strong belief in God is OK within the teaching arena as long as you do not pressure others with your convictions. Should you do so, there is the possibility that a student would complain. Should one persist in the behavior, grounds for removal are certain. Right or wrong, the first step in deletion of one's work identity has taken place when one is removed from the working environment. Once one internalizes the loss, the despair that follows may cause anger, depression, or overcompensation in some way as in John's case in church. Agoraphobia for John was the first step to demoralization, the next step the twilight zone.

The Case of Hal

Hal was also a God fearing man, but he really liked women, a lot. Hal was single so he could indulge his self to the extreme. He was no Adonis; however, he was more than acceptable in the looks department. Hal was a male nurse, and contrary to some who believe he was gay, he was very much the *ladies* man. He had a new girlfriend almost every night. On weekends when he was not on call or working, he would have several women in his company. By the time Hal was forty, he was no closer to a permanent relationship than when he was twenty. By the time he was fifty his body and looks began to fade. He had become just another person working in a hospital. The nurses that used to find him sexy had moved on to relationships, mostly marriage. Hal would take home adult movies to exercise his prostate. Eventually he ended up paying for sex with women of ill repute. Aloneness engulfed him. One morning he did not show up for work. Later that day they found him in his apartment dead by his own hand.

An example to the extreme, but a possible outcome for one who is heavily weighted in the psychochemical part of the triad. Remember that in many cases an emotional illness is nothing more than an exaggeration of the normal. Hal was so weighted in the psychochemical that his intellect and belief system were clouded. He needed help but was unable to heed his own symptoms, even though a nurse. Like the mechanic that drives a junk-heap, Hal did no upkeep on his self, body or soul.

The Case of Oscar

Oscar did not go to church. He was a self-proclaimed agnostic. However, Oscar had a PhD in psychology, and he let everyone know—to the extreme. By the time he was thirty-five he had a great teaching job. He had declined doing therapy or counseling as he felt it was just a bunch of bullshit; stating, "I don't do that touchy feely stuff."

He was one of those instructors that made one feel stupid. His students often complained that he talked down to them. After many complaints to the dean, Oscar was summoned to the dean's office for a little chat. The dean was concerned about Oscar's attitude and questioned whether he should continue teaching his present course, an introduction to psychology. Oscar proclaimed that the students wanted something for nothing, equating them with monkeys wanting bananas without doing anything to earn them. "Just a bunch of stupid brats," he said. The dean took exception to his comment stating, "We are here for them, that is the bottom line, like it, or leave it, your choice." Oscar stood, "In that case I will leave it. Besides, I have a great offer to do research, I think that I will take it, good day Sir," and left.

Oscar had no relationships with men or women. His primary relationship was gathering information, especially within the psychological realm of knowledge. His main love was his computer and book collection. In time, he became reclusive and paranoid. He published a book on introductory psychology by the time he was forty. He was invited to speak and do book signings. Evidently his book was quite good, although a little sardonic in places. His skepticism about life and God seemed to work well in the book. His paranoid view of reality caused his speaking and book signing to be short lived. Oscar became reclusive. Eventually he was the one who needed therapy.

However, this story has a happy conclusion. While in therapy, he met a wonderful and understanding woman. They eventually married. Oscar had developed a belief in something other than knowledge, a warm loving person that gave depth to his being and expanded his psyche, soma and spirit. In a word, it gave *depth* to his triad; now having existence in all three parts, he was reborn.

Time Expanding

It is obvious that life is not so cut-and-dried. Our existence in this organic reality is fleeting. One can only gather the here-and-now of being. Within the confines of the now, it is possible to reflect on the past and prepare for the future. My hope is that this information can assist one in that process.

Awareness is one's best council. Without a look into self, few of us will take the time to make changes in our behavior. The problem may be that we have no reason for an internal quest. If you have body odor, and no one tells you, will you discover for yourself that you smell? Anyone who has sat in a warm classroom with one who has that problem will tell you that it is very hard to do so. It takes courage to confront one with their aroma. Again, awareness is one's best council.

The simplistic metaphor with body odor may be too far an abstraction from the reality of personality development to be useful. One who would be aware that they smelled would have to have had an appreciation of the difference between smelling and not smelling. A behavior at this level presupposes some kind of learning. So then, what is awareness? Some call this awareness psychesthesia, an awareness that we exist. Cogito ergo sum.

Time Expanding

Catch me if you can, for I am
A most elusive guest
Existing only in your preconscious
Made of bits and pieces—
Taken from a moving stream
As each second leaps foreword
Spending time as if
It had material existence.

Hold me in your mind's-eye
Long enough to gather meaning
That I may serve you well,
Create a common bond,
Give meaning to this now
Of the mounting moment
Entwined with time expanding.

I am thought
Psychological perseverance
That determines self

An electrochemical being
Cogito ergo sum.

Awareness Times Three

Remember that old saying *me myself and I*. Perhaps there are three of us, each part having some control. Eric Berne's Transactional analysis regarding the three ego states, parent, child and adult, may have some credence. If we apply the psychespiritual, psychochemical and psychointellectual ruler to the child, adult and parent, we may find some interesting associations.

Some would say that the child is more rooted in the psychochemical world of organic reality. A step further finds an association with the psychespiritual in the parent and lastly a relevance to the adult in the psychointellectual. It would be easy if the metaphor ended there. A human personality is much more complex than limiting its existence to parent, adult, and child. As we experience life with others, we take on a bit of everyone that we contact especially intimate contact.

In a world of people, millions of people, we are but one, but it would be a mistake to believe that we make no difference. Awareness times three explicitly deals with our relationship to the world of others, and that we have an awareness of our self, our humanness, and our relationship with God, as we believe Him to be. As I stated in my personal creed, page 96, it takes courage, strength, life, love, and understanding to become actualized. The creed is a mantra that must be lived every day and one day at a time. When spoken aloud it may make give you goose bumps. Each part of the awareness times three: self, others, and God [in perception] have a powerful place in organic reality.

The Power of Self

Psychesthesia, awareness of self has many veils. The concept of Johari's[36] Window reveals more:

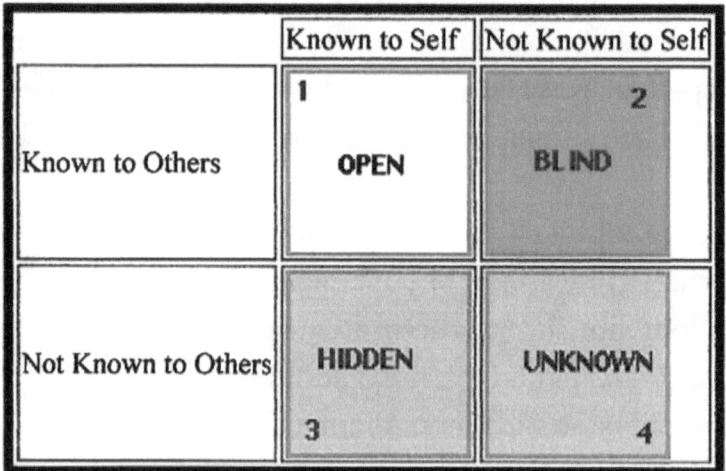

	Known to Self	Not Known to Self
Known to Others	1 OPEN	2 BLIND
Not Known to Others	HIDDEN 3	UNKNOWN 4

Quadrant 1—the area of free activity, or open area, refers to behavior and motivation known to self and known to others.

Quadrant 2—the blind area is where others can see things in ourselves of which we are unaware.

Quadrant 3—the avoided or hidden area represents things we know but do not reveal to others (e.g. a hidden agenda or matters about which we have sensitive feelings).

---

[36]   Created by Joseph Luft and Harrington Ingham in 1955.

Quadrant 4—the area of unknown activity points to the area where neither the individual nor others are aware of certain behavior motives. Yet we can assume their existence because eventually some of these things become known and we then realize that these unknown behaviors and motives were influencing relationships all along.

Quadrant 4 is of particular interest as it may include subconscious psychological information in the form of dreams. The following dream is related to show its place in communication, though with a Freudian twist.

Dream Life Related to Stages of Development

I was alone on a cobble stone street. There was a red brick building just in front of me, not more than 50 yards away. Looking out a window three floors up a woman unclad from the waist up, with pendulous breasts, waving to me, calling me to come up to her room. I next found myself in an elevator. Somehow, I was aware that she had told me that her room number was 304. I pushed the button for the third floor. When the elevator door opened, I started down the hall only to notice that I was not on the third floor but one above it. I tried several more times, but was unable to reach the right floor or room. I woke up.

Allowing the dreamer to free-associate, this possible interpretation became known. The cobblestone street, red brick building, unclad woman, third floor, the number 304, the elevator and his inability to reach the room were important symbols.

The cobblestone street identifies the time, which is long ago. For this dream, it may represent an old feeling, part of the remembrance of childhood. The red brick building that *must* be entered may represent sexual excitation. The woman with the exposed breasts may represent an infantile desire, stage, or a promise. The elevator trip up, one of further excitation; some may intimate that a higher seat of learning resides here. The number 304 may represent a homosexual latency.[37] The number three represents sexuality, the entire male genitalia, and the zero the oral stage of development. The four may be an indication that they are to be considered together. This combination may relate to the sexual outlet, which in adulthood may refer to homosexuality. However, in the dream it was impossible to reach the room, which may suggest that once you have passed through this stage successfully that you are unable to return. If so, this may confirm, for this person, that an inner conflict does exist, a confirmation only a few of us get by way of our dreams and a possible proof for the rest of us that these stages do exist. I say possible, not to make the same mistake that Freud did, we need not base a theory on one single case. With a careful case history for each individual, one can focus on the symbols that have the most meaning for that person regardless of the exogenous prattle in psychological theory. One should fit the cure to the individual, not the individual to the system.

---

[37] The sexual life, Freud finds has rich symbolism. The number three symbolizes the entire male genitalia. Mullahy, Patrick, <u>Oedipus Myth and Complex,</u> New York, Grove Press, 1955 (pg 82).

Having tunnel vision, excluding all but one system may limit understanding and self-growth. At any rate, it would be great to defrag the brain once and awhile regardless of method.

From this quadrant, poetry can also erupt. Here is another example of Freudian thinking. The unknown by analogy becomes the unconscious. It is most difficult to get away from Freudian thought. He may have given some of the best, albeit, speculative ideology on human thought/behavior. Knowing self seems to be important. Knowing self times three, most important.

The blind quadrant 2 is one that therapists work on. What is known to others, but not to ourselves, can hurt us. It is not the simplistic bad breath or spinach on our teeth; but the deep-rooted stuff that we reveal unconsciously without intent. Four conditions support the dynamic unconscious, posthypnotic phenomena, parapraxis, symptoms, and dreams. Parapraxis represents slips of the tongue, minor errors thought to reveal subconscious motives. Such as a man saying, "Oh, yeah—I was going to take my wife to the vet." What was he thinking, or better yet, what was the inference? The concept of the lie detector works on the principle that one cannot hide the truth from showing physiologically. *The truth is in there.* Anyone with a modicum of training can usually spot an untruth with ease.

Symptoms in the psychological sense may represent something of the goings-on beyond conscious awareness. Only the most deleterious usually stand out and cry for help. The more insidious ones may cause unknown harm in relationships, work routine, and one's ability to achieve. Personality aberrations often come from such hidden qualities in psychological development. The paranoid personality, a character and behavior disorder, a histrionic person or one who must always be right. While each of us has a proclivity to these traits, most of us have an awareness that we do.

Physical symptoms can also be of such origin. For years, it was believed that a stomach ulcer had to do with certain types of personality. Today we understand that these ulcers have a relationship to H pylori bacteria.

Hysterical paralysis comes to mind. Globus hystericus, the lump in the throat that will not go away when one cannot swallow what is going on in his/her life. We treat the mind to heal the body and often may treat the body to heal the mind. Keeping one's mind active with constant learning assists with the prolongation of life. What you do not use, you lose.

Warning physical symptoms may alert one of body harm or resident disease. One who smokes gets these warnings every day with a cough that is the by-product of pneumonitis. Chest pain that is not hiatial hernia brings one to a cardiologist. Low back pain can be symptomatic of disc disease or problems not related to the back at all. The mind plays an important role in sending information out—one has to learn to identify the signals.

The Landscape of Poetry[38]

Another way that one might be in touch with self is through the writing of poetry. If one thinks of poetry as reflections of our immortal soul, or at least, ripples in the waters of our deep unconscious, one may further intimate that these same ripples indicate something of the undercurrent of desires, impulses, and hidden idiosyncrasies of our personality that cry out for us to recall, spell out, or decipher. It follows then that we must view some of these self-made ripples in order to identify the underlying pressures of our own unknown. We may become better acquainted with our inner self to the degree that our mental health is improved; for, who among us can profess to know self to certainty?[39]

The Following Poem Is Given

Alterations by Time[40]

How insidious you are
Forever creeping up on me—
Making silent alterations
In the stuff, you weave so well.
What havoc have you done me?
The image in the mirror,
The wrinkled sallow skin,
The graying thinning hair.
Friend and foe-man too,
You have caught me by surprise.

---

[38] Found as an endnote.
[39] William Russell, <u>The Seduction of Time, et al</u>, Xlibris Corporation, 2004, pg 7.
[40] Ibid, pg 54.

Stolen my youth away.
But I smile a timeworn grin,
My memories live on within.

In the forgoing, a poetic catharsis exists. An awareness of growing old is common to all, but the ability to escape the psychological dilemma of *what's next*, is to some degree, prevented—a kind of psychological procrastination. The poem deals symbolically with the process of aging in a healing way. Self-awareness in this instant puts off thinking about the infinity of death by recalling the past memories of life.

The Power of Others

I am too what others think. In as much as I am my own person, I am often caused to act in a way known to others. Upon meeting a new acquaintance, I can be whomever I want. Upon meeting a known acquaintance, I must choose to be that person known to him/her. Expectations by parents for their children often hamper their life-choices. This awareness is known by anyone who wanted to be an artist, while their parent(s) expected them to become a doctor, lawyer, or whatever. Therefore, an awareness of who you are as thought by others may be an important factor in caused behavior.

I often think of type casting. I once played a doctor in a play. From that time on, I was often considered for roles that carried a medical persona. In life, one may play a role, be in a role, or wish for a role. Your awareness of your role in life may be as important as the part you think you play. Your choice is to make the role you play real, or change the role others have cast upon you and become the role of your choice.

The Power of God [in perception]

The third part of self-awareness times three is the most difficult to be in touch with. While it may be self-evident for some that one should believe, it may be just as self-evident to others that belief in God is human, but nothing more. I have chosen the words *in perception* so as not to offend. Right or wrong, behavior will give clue to a person's primary belief system. You can go to church on Sunday and then raise hell the rest of the week. Or, you can do the opposite. Behavior will speak for you long before anyone takes the time to evaluate what you believe.

I spent a year in Vietnam as a medic. I do not recall one man dieing that denied God. In one instant, a man with his last breath looked into space with a smile stating, "Wow!" then closed eyes in deaths slumber. Up to that time, I may have had my doubts, but no more. This is what makes it so important that one is in touch with their belief about God. As in the poem, alterations by time, you can put off the inevitable in thought process, but not in actuality. None of us get out of this world alive. From this conclusion, one must choose how they want to live. I have chosen to teach and to heal. Read aloud my personal creed once more. Better yet, copy it onto another paper and read it every day. It is impossible to be an anus equinus after having done so for at least an hour.

The Power of God [in prayer]

If you are one who has chosen to believe, then this portion is for you, the rest of you can skip this section. Einstein may have spoken of God in the abstract when he brought forth his theory of relativity. Time, motion, gravitation are all products of the universe of God. Some would say that God is infinite, the eternal logos. Others posit that God is humankind in totality, each one of us part of the whole that is God. If you take away one person, you take something from all of us. If you give to the whole, you give to yourself. The golden rule is a product of this kind of thought. The worship of God has matured over the centuries from a matriarchal to the present patriarchal form; from idol worship to one belief found in the person of Jesus. A form of prayer probably has been used to talk to the unseen forces since humankind developed voice. The documentation of what prayer can achieve is voluminous.

If you believe in prayer as healer, as gift giver, as forgiver, and as the way to achieve fulfillment, then you believe in something greater than self. The primary weakness in any belief of this nature is that we can tell you to believe, but the proof lies within the person; it is not a material thing put to a physical test per se. In the moment of true prayer, one *knows* in a way that cannot be tested by physical laws; yet, it is part of the material reality we call now. In prayer, there exists a place where time does not persist. There have been numerous examples of this in stories about group prayer where time and space changed, in some way, to the surprise of the persons involved. Prayer heals, binds time, and strengthens our connection to the God of our choice.

Belief Models to Organic/Nonorganic Reality

1. Medical Model—The medical model entails all that we know about the body through medical science. We act in a universe of viruses, bacterium, and diseases of the body that we combat with chemicals, drugs, and operations. It is a world in which the cure is often as dangerous as the disease or malady, and a world in which the diseases are slowly overtaking us. However, in the new world of the computer we shall take back our territory, and once again make headway to out distant the onslaught of the microbe.

2. The Alternative Health Model—Perhaps more primitive, but no less important, are the models that include homeopathic, herbal remedies, acupuncture, massage, and a number of ways to heal the body that do not include the newborn chemicals and scientific advances of today.

3. Models of Mind—There are personality theories that include psychoanalysis, behaviorism, humanism, general semantics, self-actualization, rational-emotive theory, and a host of theories too long to include.

The forgoing represents a brief sketch into human thought. An individual works in the world, as he believes it to be, the model that is used becomes a way of life. Problems solved and changes in behavior are consonant with the components of belief. A person will see the world in an expected way. It is the old story that when you give a child a hammer for his birthday, he will find many things to hammer.

EDUCATION'S FINAL PLUNGE

Looking to the Future

As is always the case, things change. It so happens that in education much changes, and often not always for the betterment of the students. As I write this addendum, I am taking a different direction in life. My reason, in part, follows.

One of the reasons that I decided that changing to an online course was a poor idea had to do with the faltering condition of the distant learning course I was teaching. In the past, for each semester, I would write a summary of the course for the powers-that-be. It was obvious to me that the distant learning course I was presently teaching, in preparation to an online course, had its share of shortcomings. I had put hours of work into the course, CD creation, my book, and a complete syllabus, shown earlier. However, it was not enough. Although the following summary is without negative comments by the students, it does not give a good evaluation when you compare it with past classes.

Summary for Medical Terminology

SUBJECT: Summary for Distant Learning
Medical Terminology

TO: Dean of Instruction

FROM: William J. Russell, Part-Time Instructor

METHODOLOGY & PRESENTATION:

1. 11 chapters covered in the book *Medical Terminology by the Mnemonic Story System.*

2. Information CD's covering chapters 2 thru 11 can be purchased in the college bookstore.

3. 4 meetings of a maximum of 3 hours each and a final are required, and Three tests each given at the beginning of the hour with a final given in the last three hours.

4. Lecture and discussion is dependent on the time left after each test.
    Lecture format on CD for the following:

    a. Orthopaedic conditions,
    b. Pharmacology,
    c. Neuropsychiatric conditions, mainly schizophrenia, and
    d. Communication theory.

5. A film on orthopaedic surgery if time allows.

RESULTS OF CLASS PERFORMANCE:

Students	Fall Semester 2007 Distant Learning	Spring Semester 2007 Distant Learning
Signed up	36	17
Did not start—drop later	09	06
Dropped—all	11	07
Completed	10	06
Incomplete	03	00
Failed	09 Due to not dropping class	02 Due to not dropping class

See legend below:

Signed up: Although 36 signed up, only 26 showed up for the orientation, and, for the first test 16 appeared and the second test only 12, for the third test 9 and the final 10. If all the incomplete students make up their work, it may become 13 students completing the course.

Did not Start: Nine students did not start and of these four later dropped.

Dropped: Eleven dropped, most of them early. A few of them did appear for one or two tests, but then failed to continue. I was not notified of their reasons for discontinuing the course.

Completed: Ten completed the course with an A grade. Interesting to note, on the story part of the final exam, nine students got a 100% and one 80%. This part of the final is what the mnemonic story system is all about.

Incomplete: Three students failed to take the final. Letters will be sent, but there is a section of the syllabus that tells them what they should do.

GRADE STATISTICS:

Year	Fall 2007	Spring 2007
Mean[41]	**96.7**	**88.9**
S. Deviation[42]	**4.57**	**9.79**

COMMENTS/RECOMMENDATIONS/CONCERNS BY INSTRUCTOR:

1. This is the second class offered as a distant learning CD class for medical terminology.

2. I have little to offer here, as I have been told that this class will be going to an online status. The only question that I have is this, is it because this class falls under the rubric of business office technology? Or, will many other part time employees be given the same direction for their courses?

3. Having taught medical terminology over 21 years it is my dutiful conviction that much will be lost. I can only hope that I do not have to give tests online as well, that would be a disaster.

---

[41] Based on the score obtained on the final before bonus points are included.
[42] ibid

COMMENTS BY STUDENTS;

Comments from final copied verbatim:

1. Thank you, and the word association does work, I wasn't sure at the beginning of the class, but it worked. Thank you.

2. I really enjoyed your class and I learned a lot of useful terms that I will keep with me as I go on to my career. Thank you.

3. I listened to the lectures (on CD) about 3 times each. They were very interesting but way over my head. I apologize for not doing better on this section of the test. The problem I assure you is all mine. I just don't have the background yet to understand it all. But thanks.

4. Thank you for stretching our brains and for the creative style of mnemonics. It is obvious that the time and care you took in creating this format was driven by passion. The passion you had to ensure your students success in learning and most importantly, retaining what they have learned. Keep up the forward momentum and stay well.[43]

CLASS SCHEDULE DESCRIPTION:

Give yourself the power of understanding and using medical terminology. When your doctor says, "The patient must refrain

---

[43] These comments by students are available for inspection, should anyone feel the need to see. This was never asked for in all the years I taught at Mendocino Community College, Ukiah, California.

from heterosexual interdigitation." You can say, "Is that so the dactylitis won't become dactylosymphysis?" Enroll in medical terminology today!

TEXT:

Russell, William. <u>Medical Terminology by the Mnemonic Story System,</u> Xlibris Corporation, 1st edition, 2006.

CLOSING STATEMENT: (For last class taught)

Like feathers torn from a pillow in high wind, are words once spoken, never to be reclaimed, lost in the indelible memory of time. I know, for I have written and spoken a few. For me, some have been too harsh, even though a modicum of truth at times prevailed. I cannot take them back, but I can apologize, consider it so. Sometimes the wounds of truth persist, and pain the most, for those whose psychological selectivity has given rise to meanings not intended.

I would like to thank you for the many years of help and the words of kindness you have expressed. Although dutiful, your words on my many evaluations have been thoughtful and kindly received. I am thankful for the twenty years that I have had, and I will remember them with kind regard. They say that when one door closes, another will open; I hope that is true for I am not ready to give in to nothingness.

Thank you for allowing me to direct this course. If I can be of any further assistance, please contact me by e-mail: willirusse7@aol.com.

Meaning Point:

With classroom time reduced, the responsibility for learning weighs heavy upon the student. It is important to have a text, syllabus and CD or video collection that support the lectures giving the effect of increased time in the classroom. The simple educational concept of verbal repetition is not enough.

APPENDIX—ENDNOTES

ENDNOTE 1

Education—Primary Discourse

Cyberspaces

Let us gather up some sleepless nights
With online visitations in hasty flights
Found in an infinity of cyberspaces
Complete with bloodless places
Classrooms without a human touch
Instructors that care not much
Where instruction shown upon a faceless screen
On a computer that can hear no scream
While powers-that-be sleep without remorse
For the damage done by each online course
Where rooms with four corners are forever lost
While students do not realize the dreadful cost
   So long as these courses exist online
   That long we set back learning in time

The following essay I wrote at the time that I was informed that my class was to become an online course. I believe that I irritated one dean to the point of my extinction. I was not offered to teach the course the next semester with an indication that I would be put on a list since *they* needed to broaden their selection process. I was never offered the course again. However, this does not change my view. I had 21 years teaching medical terminology, perhaps it was time for someone else to get the opportunity.

Vanishing Classrooms

There is a ubiquitous cloud that is about to befall us. No one seems to care. Learning is about to be dealt a blow so severe that all but a few classrooms will be left. This oncoming tidal wave is in the form of online education; a bloodless form of learning so simplistically seductive that the danger remains hidden from view.

With our present education system, wallowing in the mud of imperfection, the chosen way of least resistance is online teaching. The classroom size will dwindle until only the powerful computer shall stand, cold, bloodless, and impervious to human thought or question. We need to get back to some of the ways of yesteryear, a philosophical backward glance of the not too long ago.

Sometime in 1976, I wrote what I called then, *My Personal Creed*. Over the years, it has been revisited by many different names: *A Nurses Prayer, A Mantra for Living* to name a few (Chapter 9).

The creed now updated, with paragraph 6, a place with four corners called a room.

6. *Give me a place where I can touch the lives of those in quest of knowledge with communication. A place with four corners called a room. Learning should take place with a breathing, feeling person that can provide feedback; let me be that someone. Human thought is done best when shared with another face to face.*

ENDNOTE 2

Education—Continuing Discourse

Downsizing Education
One Class at a Time

It should be a fundamental right for every student to spend some of their time in a classroom. However, for some subjects the classroom is most important; one such subject is medical terminology. Changing a medical terminology course from 51 hours to 15 hours is like trying to teach someone to swim in a bathtub, you'll get wet, but little else. For medical terminology, distant learning is that bathtub. Changing a course is even more likely to happen to you if you are a part time instructor.

Today many community colleges find it easy to enlist workers part time. Often this means that instructors have no guarantee regarding their ongoing employment. They must succumb to the dictates of circumstance. In the education arena, especially community colleges, this is very much the situation. Part time employees have little to say regarding their class beyond the actual presentation of material. Therefore, if the *powers-that-be* decide to change the course, delete the course, or alter the way the course is taught, the instructor is bound to comply. Having said this, one can guess what effect this must have on student learning capability when only given the opportunity to take a class by video or another option under the umbrella of distant learning.

Distant learning may bring with it a propensity for one to cheat, parrot back information, and to become an automaton of information, a reflection of the work on the printed page; alas, a bloodless substitute for the reality it purports to portray. Learning should take place in a room with a breathing, feeling person that can provide feedback. After all, isn't that what communication is about, an interchange of ideas between language users capable of sharing feelings, stories, ideas and a host of attributes too long to list. Knowledge cannot exist in a vacuum. Human thought is best when shared with another. Some courses will never lend themselves to a distant learning process.

If we do not take a stand now, when the time comes for our demise, especially as classroom instructors, there will be no one left to stand, the classroom will be bare.

ENDNOTE 3

Education—Continuing Discourse

The Last Refuge of a Free Society

That which we developed last may often be what we lose first. This holds true when we are challenged physically, spiritually, or emotionally. However, the most insidious of all may be something as simple as the loss created by an innovation; the computer. Putting language down on something concrete, like a book, gives man permanence in time. Putting language in cyberspace is an infinite insanity, and may be our *tower of babble.*

There have been times in our history when books were burned. These inflictions upon our written language were obvious—classrooms in cyberspace are not. The last refuge of a free society is the collection of knowledge stored in libraries and our freedom to go there with human touch, and blow away the dust of time from a volume of our choice; or to a class, in a room, of our choice.

Education is a two-way street, you listen and you read. Then, you speak and you write. The communication channel is person-to-person allowing for an in-person clarification. The process may allow for the computer, but the dynamics of learning must include personal contact. If the computer becomes all, we lose the affect in communication, and the soul of understanding.

If the computer is the way of the future in education, then we need to modify its use in the classroom. Online classes threaten to engulf the education process. It is necessary to limit these courses and to instill some control measures to ensure honesty and integrity in the ongoing education system. Should we fail, the onslaught of online courses could jeopardize the degree system and cause further failures in education.

Our academic freedom to teach within the confines of a classroom may be the next freedom to fall. When an instructor is forced to teach a class online, or not to teach at all, the line has been drawn; academic freedom has begun to atrophy. Where once we had a place with four corners, we now have an infinite space. It is not wrong to have access to cyberspace, but it is wrong to dictate how a course is to be taught. It is more wrong, when the powers-that-be are challenged, to have more than one course of the same genre taught online just so an instructor cannot teach in a classroom; even more wrong to deny students a place in a classroom for that same course. It is not logical to assume that all students want to learn online.

It is time for all the instructors that have lost their freedom to teach in a classroom to make their voice heard. Or, like sheep to the slaughter, let come what may.

ENDNOTE 4

Education—Suggestion

Back to the Drawing Board
(Previously printed material has been included for
continuity in this article)

*The following outline in lesson plan format describes the
organization of this paper.*

I. **Introduction:**
    A. Opening Statement: For the longest . . . .
    B. Read: The teacher Talks to the Student

II. **Explanation:**
    A. Student evaluations of teachers as part of the teacher's
        evaluation.
        1. High and low evaluations.
        2. Compare with student's grade.
        3. How often done.

    B. Evaluation of course/curriculum.
        1. Lesson plans.
        2. Book/text

    C. Teacher's evaluations.
        1. By staff.
        2. By self.

D. Evaluation of course.
1. Summary.
2. Comments on summary.

III. **Closing Statement:**

There, you have it, the process of evaluation both ways; of the instructor and by the instructor. In all fairness, to allow the students to have a dominate say about instruction is quite dangerous. There is one other thing that I must include, as it has to do with online courses, and it shall be the last entry of this paper

---

Introduction:

For the longest time, there has been an ongoing argument about student evaluations being part of the teacher's evaluation. Regardless of how one feels about this, it seems logical that there should be a method to this madness. What I propose in this paper may be some ways to soften the blow.

Explanation:

Student Evaluations of Teachers:

It is a known fact that a student doing poorly in a subject may tend to blame the teacher while a student doing well might praise the teacher.

To offset this it is suggested that of the battery of evaluations turned in by any class of students, the top five percent and bottom five percent be eliminated.

It would be a good idea to have these evaluations done once a year for each subject taught.

Evaluations of Course/Curriculum:

Each course taught should have a lesson plan on file. Obviously, a text from which to teach is necessary for most subjects, and a desirable asset; especially, if one uses an outline or lesson plan to support the text. Using a text requires periodic updates to be sure information is current. During an evaluation by a peer the text should be available as an evaluation of how the text is used; and is an important part of the teacher's evaluation.

Teachers Evaluation of Staff/Self:

By Staff:

Some questions that staff should consider

1. Knowledge of subject.
2. Communication ability.
3. Student interaction.
4. Course organization and materials
5. Understandability of subject.
6. Use of handouts, etc.

Each school will have their preference.

By Self:

1. Why do you teach/subject?
2. Who is your favorite author (explicit for course taught)?
3. What is a best student/worst?
4. What is your best day teaching/worst?

Over the years, I have asked students about their philosophies in 500 words or less. I am thinking, that maybe it is a good question for an instructor. Along with a philosophy, a person should have a belief model on how the world is. This is a good question.

Evaluation of Course by Instructor:

In order to keep one abreast of oneself and in tune with reality, I suggest that each instructor provide a summary for the powers-that-be by producing a document that summarizes the course just taught. An example follows:

SUBJECT: Summary for Distant Learning
            Medical Terminology

TO: _____

FROM: William J. Russell, Part-Time Instructor

METHODOLOGY & PRESENTATION:

1. 11 chapters covered in the book *Medical Terminology by the Mnemonic Story System.*

2. Information CD's covering chapters 2 thru 11 can be purchased in the college bookstore.

3. 4 meetings of a maximum of 3 hours each and a final are required. 3 tests each given at the beginning of the hour, for a total of 4 tests.

4. Lecture and discussion is dependent on the time left after each test.
   Lecture format on CD for the following:

   a. Orthopaedic conditions,
   b. Pharmacology, and
   c. Neuropsychiatric conditions, mainly schizophrenia.
   d. Communication theory.

RESULTS OF CLASS PERFORMANCE:

Students	Fall Semester 2007 Distant Learning	Spring Semester 2007 Distant Learning
Signed up	36	17
Did not start—drop later	09	06
Dropped—all	11	07
Completed	10	06

Incomplete	03	00
Failed	09 Due to not dropping class	02 Due to not dropping class

See legend below:

Signed up: Although 36 signed up, only 26 showed up for the orientation, and, for the first test, 16 appeared and the second test only 12, for the third test 9 and the final 10. If all the incomplete students make up their work, it may become 13 students completing the course.

Did not Start: Nine students did not start and of these four later dropped.

Dropped: Eleven dropped, most of them early. A few of them did appear for one or two tests, but then failed to continue. I was not notified either by phone or in writing for their reasons for not continuing the course.

Completed: Ten completed the course with an A grade. Interesting to note, on the story part of the final exam, nine students got a 100% and one 80%. This part of the final is what the mnemonic story system is all about.

Incomplete: Three students failed to take the final. Letters will be sent, but there is a section of the syllabus that tells them what they should do.

GRADE STATISTICS:

Year	Fall 2007	Spring 2007
Mean[44]	**96.7**	**88.9**
S. Deviation[45]	**4.57**	**9.79**

COMMENTS/RECOMMENDATIONS/CONCERNS BY INSTRUCTOR:

1. This is the second class offered as a distant learning CD class for medical terminology.

2. I have little to offer here, as I have been told that this class will be going to online status. The only question that I have is this, is it because this class falls under the rubric of business office technology? Or, will many other part time employees be given the same direction for their courses?

3. Having taught medical terminology since 1974, it is my dutiful conviction that much will be lost. I can only hope that I do not have to give tests online as well, that would be a disaster.

COMMENTS BY STUDENTS:

Comments from final copied verbatim:

1. Thank you, and the word association does work, I wasn't sure at the beginning of the class, but it worked. Thank you.

---

[44] Based on the score obtained on the final before bonus points are included.
[45] ibid

2. I really enjoyed your class and I learned a lot of useful terms that I will keep with me as I go on to my career. Thank you.

3. I listened to the lectures (on CD) about 3 times each. They were very interesting but way over my head. I apologize for not doing better on this section of the test. The problem I assure you is all mine. I just don't have the background yet to understand it all. But thanks.

4. Thank you for stretching our brains and for the creative style of mnemonics. It is obvious that the time and care you took in creating this format was driven by passion. The passion you had to ensure your students success in learning and most importantly, retaining what they have learned. Keep up the forward momentum and stay well.[46]

CLASS SCHEDULE DESCRIPTION:

Give yourself the power of understanding and using medical terminology. When your doctor says, "The patient must refrain from heterosexual interdigitation." You can say, "Is that so the dactylitis won't become dactylosymphysis?" Enroll in medical terminology today!

TEXT:

Russell, William. *Medical Terminology by the Mnemonic Story System.* Xlibris Corporation, 1st edition, 2006.

---

[46] These comments by students are available for inspection, should anyone feel the need to see. In the 21 years at Mendocino College, Ukiah, California-Regrettably, I was never asked.

CLOSING STATEMENT:

Thank you for allowing me to *direct* this course. If I can be of any further assistance, please contact me by e-mail: willirusse7@aol.com or phone 463-0892.

Sincerely,

William J. Russell

Act to limit online classes

Online classes threaten to engulf the educational arena. It is necessary to limit these courses and to instill some control measures to ensure honesty and integrity to the ongoing education system. Should we fail, the onslaught of online courses could jeopardize the degree system and cause further failures in a system already fragile.

1. Online courses should comprise 45% of all courses taught that qualify as academic. Additionally, to be cost effective, the pay schedule for instructors teaching online should be adjusted so that greed does not infect the process. This excludes courses not taught in a conventional classroom.

2. A classroom defined as—*Give me a place where I can touch the lives of those in quest of knowledge with communication. A place with four corners called a room. Learning should take place with a breathing, feeling person that can provide feedback.*

3. Online courses should have the final exam given in a place where the person taking the exam is physically present. Obviously, this is for the reason of honesty. When online, how can you be sure the person taking the exam is the student and not a friend with knowledge in the subject?

4. Classroom courses should comprise 55% of the classes offered by any community college. The maintenance of the

education process depends on the interaction of student to instructor face to face.

5. No instructor shall be caused to teach his/her class on line arbitrarily. Any such decision should include the instructor's input. An instructor shall not be denied teaching in a classroom just so a class can be taught online unless the instructor is given his/her say. This should be especially true for classroom courses that have been taught successfully for three or more semesters. When in contention, an academic committee and/or faculty committee should intervene allowing the instructor to present reasons why the class should remain as taught.

6. Online courses should demonstrate balance. At least one classroom course should be available in the event that there are students that cannot take a particular course online. There is the fact that some colleges will probably have learning centers with many computers that will allow many to learn, with assistance, online. It is our future.

[Final] Closing Statement:

Today, like no other time, we are faced with the possibility of losing our place in the world of knowledge. As we struggle to stay afloat, we are damaging our educational process by forcing many teachers to teach online. Let us be realistic, we need teachers, instructor, and educators of all kind and in all fields.

If we are going to allow the evaluation process, by students, to be the primary focus, and the online course to dominate our curriculum, we had better take another look. Back to the drawing board is my contribution. Think about it.

ENDNOTE 5

Education—Proposal for Distant Learning Class

Vice President of Academic Affairs
Mendocino Community College
1000 Hensley Drive
Ukiah, CA 95482

Dear Dean,

This letter is to introduce you to the proposal regarding medical terminology for a distant learning project. The following proposal shall explain what I plan to do to create a course in a distant learning format.

Sincerely,

William J. Russell
Part time instructor

Medical Terminology for Distant Communication

Based on the book

Medical Terminology
by the
Mnemonic Story System[47]

Proposal Summary:

Eleven videos made to accompany the book, *Medical Terminology by the Mnemonic Story System*. Each chapter covered by one video. Videos should be no longer than two hours with a mean of 1.5 hours. All material that the student will need for the course is within the book and videos. A student, after the orientation period, might be able to complete the course using only the book. However, it will not be recommended that a student should do so. The videos will contain all the information that the student will need to take the three tests and one final examination. A book is included so that you can inspect the contents.

---

[47]   To be published by Xlibris

PROPOSAL

I   INTRODUCTION:

1. Using a classroom, I shall make eleven videos.

2. The book, along with the videos, will be *Medical Terminology by the Mnemonic Story System.*

3. Chapters:
  a. One, A Beginning in Word Recognition
  b. Two, Mnemonics, ab—to cantho—
  c. Three, Mnemonics, capit—to cut—
  d. Four, Mnemonics, cyan—to ex—
  e. Five, Mnemonics, fascia to hypno—
  f. Six, Mnemonics, hypo—to—malacia
  g. Seven, Mnemonics, malign—to onych—
  h. Eight, Mnemonics, oophor—to phot—
  i. Nine, Mnemonics, phragma—to radic—
  j. Ten, Mnemonics, ramus to strict—
  k. Eleven, Mnemonics, sub—to—vulse

4. Schedule for Classes: (one month apart)
  a. Saturday   9AM to Noon Orientation/Lecture/Discussion
  b. Saturday   9AM to Noon Test first four chapters, 100 words
  c. Saturday   9AM to Noon Test second 100 words
  d. Saturday   9AM to Noon Test third 100 words
  e. Saturday   9AM to Noon Final Exam/ 90 words plus story

5. With each 100 words of all tests will be a story that is practice. On the final, the story will count as 10% of test grade.

6. At the orientation there will be given additional handouts that will assist the students with the course due to the limited time that they will have with the instructor. The instructor will be available by email at <u>MnemonicBooks@ aol.com</u>.

7. There will be at least two outside classroom assignments as research papers.

II Cost of Production:

1. The only cost incurred should be the cost of the videos. All other equipment is available.

2. Time will not be a factor unless I can get no one to assist with the camera. My guess is that I may be able to ask a student with this, if the school allows. If not I may have to hire someone or ask a friend to assist.

III Conclusion:

I have used the text *Medical Terminology by the Mnemonic Story System* for many years. With the additional handouts, videos, and time in the classroom the students should get a better than average look at the subject of medical terminology. I will make myself available as is necessary so that no student will come to the end of the course empty.

I would like to thank you in advance for consideration of this proposal.

Sincerely,

William J. Russell
Part time Instructor

ENDNOTE 6

Communication

Reaching Into Self
The Landscape of Poetry

Poetry, to me, is a language all its own; a symbolic tool that can be used to vent, in an abstract way, the internal anxieties, fears, and desires of the living of life. It is an expression of me as I am this instant. Using words, a language created by others, but putting words together in a special way that speaks for me alone.

Poetry is a form of escape, a grasp at sanity or insanity, a way to unleash a verbal turmoil in an accepted way (in our society). I may formulate problems, spin them around in my mind, even sleep with them, then behold—a poem is born. If I do this, then so must others.

Verse, then, is a way for man to speak of the realities for which no concrete referent exists. A way to capture a quality about something that words alone can seldom declare.

Poetry is an impression of the very act of living. It is another way for man to raise up on his hind feet and howl at the moon or to vent his painful separation from nature in cries and moans, to make love in speaking, and finally, to speak about his end and risk a guess at what eternity must hold; in all, a noble task.

Poet, Heal thyself

Sometimes the wounds of truth persist, and pain the most, for those whose psychological selectivity has given rise. With these words, we begin a journey looking into the psychoanalytical quality of poetry, and to the quality of self-healing, it can render.

Time Expanding

Catch me if you can, for I am
A most elusive guest
Existing only in your preconscious
Made of bits and pieces—
Taken from a moving stream
As each second leaps foreword
Spending time as if
It had material existence.

Hold me in your mind's-eye
Long enough to gather meaning
That I may serve you well,
Create a common bond,
Give meaning to this now
Of the mounting moment
Entwined with time expanding.

I am thought,
Psychological perseverance
That determines self
An electrochemical being
Cogito ergo sum.[48]

The forgoing poem brings to mind the four corners of the teaching room, *perseverance, preparation, perspiration, and prayer*. These qualities must exist for a poet/writer/teacher to continue in time. Each poem that one writes gives lead to a kind of emotional catharsis. For some this can be so powerful that healing of the psyche may take place.

Poetry therapy has been around for a long time. An excellent book, "Poetry the Healer," by Jack J. Leedy, M.D., 1973, gives more than enough information for one to begin to understand and research their own work.

My purpose here is to reveal my thinking for some of the poems that I have written. Long after I cease to exist, and if these poems remain, there may be questions that readers might ask. I offer some insights and revelations.

Along with these insights, I hope to choose the poems that I believe give the most relief i.e., provoke the most change. After all, understanding at the superficial verbal level does not always bring relief. Sometimes psychological selectivity, in our writing poetry, chooses that which will heal us the most. Moreover,

---

[48]   "What I Do," Xlibris, 2008, Editors Choice Award 2007, Poetry.com. This book replaces *What I Do.*

this healing comes from a much deeper level; some say the unconscious level. It is a process of psychoanalytic healing without a therapist.

Many poems may speak for themselves. I have developed two sections. Each section or group of poems speaks to a different part of the personality. When it is necessary, I shall Meta-communicate delving into my thoughts regarding meaning.

Group One
Poems Taken From Med-Term Lectures

I have taught medical terminology for more than 35 years. In the process of getting the students attention on that first day, I used various opening statements that I hoped would grab their attention. Several follow.

The first one introduces a chapter regarding DNA and the nature of our cells.

> "What evil lurks in the genes of man?"
> This—horrible imprinting
> That seeks to corrupt by insidious intent.
> What tragedy of DNA lies hidden?
> Beneath the surface of normality?
> What latent truth will soma at last reflect—
> Only time will tell?

The second one speaks for itself.

> A suffix may an ending be,
> The last to come in a
> Words meaning tree—
> But, suffice it to say,
> Without its branching hue,
> Less meaning for me,
> And little for you.

The third entry relates to being overweight. If there is any redeeming quality to this one, it has to do with the process of rationalizing, and perhaps a little intellectualizing. Sound familiar?

> Food, the final frontier
> We are the gatherers
> Of inner space gastronome
> Our mission, to gather calories
> To explore new waist lands
> To find mirth in our girth, and
> To boldly go, where no size,
> Has gone before.

Fourth introduces the chapter on the urinary system. In an Emily Dickenson style, speaks beyond the written word. The poem may carry some healing qualities by symbol.

The sea, like our internal being
Has tides that swell,
High and low—
The sea, like love
Has peaks and valleys,
Ups and downs—
The sea, like time
Pervades the soul into eternity—
And, our internal tides
Salty brine, in kind,
From whence we came.

The fifth is more prose than poetry. If you guessed pharmacology, you would be right.

Aesculapius held down his staff,
caduceus glimmering in the sunlight,
pointing earthward; and, in a thunderous
voice spoke, "take thou as directed," and thus,
the beginning of prescriptive medicine.

Group Two
Poems from the book
The Seduction of Time, et al

The first poem in this book, *The Seduction of Time,* tells a story. When read aloud it may produce goose bumps in some. It may bring us in touch with a primitive recall, almost as deep as an olfactory memory. In this way, it may provide a cathartic release without identifying the causative agent. Alluding to the virginity of time is both interesting and audacious; that man can have his way with time is certainly Freudian. In the end man proceeds to do to himself in reality that which he has so far only proclaimed with words, the aftermath of which is infinity. In essence, screw himself, and so infinity is bound to creation, an aftermath indeed. This poem is a form of self-communication, touching the very soul of being.

The Seduction of Time

Eternal is the pressure
Of knowledge,
Fastening itself to an idea,
Clinging there, waiting
For man to discover
What he has
Known all along.

Everlasting in the force
That bathes
The brain of man,
Nourishing a notion,
Bringing to light

A spark of genius.
The gift that
Emerges in momentary
Glory from the dust of dormancy.

Never-ending is the ebb
Of time, playing
On the consciousness
Of man
Creating immortality through man
With language
Erupting from his throat of flesh
Bringing light to
Human thought.

Up from the fundament
Of the soul—
Time losing her virginity
To man,
That upstart,
Who must conquer all;
Then, with his greatest
And last triumph,
Man finally proceeds to

Do to himself in reality
What he has so far only
Proclaimed with words,
The aftermath of which
Is infinity.

The next poem, *His Myth and Seed,* on page 20 speaks to the fact that we die. Again, if anything, it speaks to the time gathering quality of language.

The inherent danger that may exist today is that we may have come so far away from reading books, that the impersonal computer may take front stage. Anyway, here is the poem.

His Myth and Seed

In all that man must feel,
And in all that man must do.
It must certainly be true
That he binds the two,
The feeling and the deed,
Together with his word,
And so perpetuates himself
With myth and seed,
Until he has met his organic
End indeed.
But this end is only
The beginning,
For his myth and seed
Will carry on the deed.

Poetry too, has the capability of rendering understanding by using language compression to any subject. Mental illness is such a subject.

Schizophrenic Places

Let us gather up some sleepless nights
With paranoid visitations in hasty flights
Found in schizophrenic places
Complete with haunted faces
Demonic dungeons in tissue abide
On faceless neurons of minds tongue-tied
Where delusions play upon a tortured soul
Ranting their soundless rasp of malcontent
While therapies pointlessly interrogate
To understand a chemistry with words
Where words—at best—collide with words
While therapies insult and insinuate
So long as disease must here reside
That long their words not reach inside

Poetry can be a self-internship into your very own subconscious, and therefore, a kind of healing process that allows you to cool an emotional hot spot. When thinking of poetry as healer, or having to do with your subconscious, it sounds as if you are talking about a form of psychoanalysis. In some small way, that may be correct. When writing poetry, it is possible that we will be bringing hidden thoughts to our conscious surface. The unknown thought process might allow one to cool that emotional hot spot. If we write about things that bother us, in metaphor, it might be that this form of abstracting may cause a lessening of anxiety. Like the speck of grit that causes a pearl in an oyster shell, our poem becomes a creation of beauty and catharsis; a process that may reveal an insight, feeling, or a new look at an old worry. The following poem creates an insight and gives one a feeling of purpose.

You Are the Seed of Now

You are what you bring to this moment,
Beyond the organic,
Very much the incalculable
Substance of being,
And in the process of being,
All that has gone before,
In whatever form,
And possibly all that will ever be (you)
You are the seed of now,
Germinating into tomorrow,
Maybe into forever.
You are a finite whisper
Within the great still—
Acoustics of the mind that only
The imagination can conjure.
You are the product of divine intervention,
Born with a soul, a body, and a purpose.
Define this purpose
And live forever;
Or cloud this purpose with doubt
And cease to exist, for then,

The viscosity of time shall
Engulf you without a single sound,
Gasp or whisper of evidence
That you ever existed at all!

Looking at love through the optic nerve of poetry may reveal subliminal desires, wishes, and ways to cope; but, the result is most always a healthy reflection, albeit—sometimes a sad one.

Chariot Revisited[49]

Because I could not stop for love,
She lustily stopped for me,
The moment held us two
And immortality.

We barely moved, she knew no haste,
And I had put away
My past and future too
For her reality.

We flew together where few have been,
Beyond this earthly place;
We passed the seas of shining blue,
We passed the setting sun.

---

[49]　This is written in the style of Emily Dickinson, ref. *The Complete Poems of,* 1960, pg 350, poem 712.

We paused before the edge of time,
At the acme of our swell;
Returning then, to dust we came,
Organic bodies homely spun.

Since then it seems a lifetime,
But each touch of her,
It seems to me,
Gives a glimpse of eternity.

Or, this one:

Love Silently or Not at All

To love aloud is very foolish,
But foolish more, I know,
To hold within the heart
A burning need to flow.

Who love, and others do not see,
Who hurt, and none observe,
Whose loving eyes no lover
Returns with burning gaze?
To love alone is very safe,
But safer more, I know,
To never loved at all,
For then, no pain to show.

And, in the heat of passion:

Ecstasy

I like a look of passion
Because I know it's true;
Men do not fake tumescence,
Nor simulate a semen flow.

The eyes with blank stare gaze,
And this is petit mort,
Impossible to sham;
Wet droplets upon the body clung,
By heated fervor flung.

Sweet daggers passion dipped,
Into entrails embedded,
Tasting nectar of love composed;
Two chemistries entwined,
Exploding, mixing timeless souls.[50]

Finally, in humor poetry defines an escape from reality, or at least an unexpected outcome of thought. From a theoretical point of view, humor can take several forms. Laughing at one who makes mistakes is a socially accepted way of suppressing unacceptable behavior. An example as with sexual jokes where the results of the joke or experience are incongruent—where the brain's processing of information leads to a resolution that produces a sense of amusement; and, playfulness that allows

---

[50]   Murder in C-Minor by W.J.Russell, 2007, Publish America, last 5 lines.

the person to see the humorous parts of life or cause laughter in others. It is often stated that the perception of humor indicates one's ability to abstract from life's experience, to be able to go beyond the concrete. By the way, concreteness often points to a personality disorder at the most and poor communication skills at the least. However, some also say that if one misses the humor in a joke, it may only be that it does not relate to his life in anyway, and therefore may have no meaning. Humor may well define personality type.

OK Croquet

A sideward glance with squinted eye,
A crack of sound, when
object round, let fly.
A shout, a moan, when
past the hoop
The ball has flown.
But only a game, play we,
Our mind, for the moment, free;
You see, it's all OK,
The game we play is, not life, per se.
Just croquet.

Or another:

Murphy's Law in Retrospect

When things seem to be going right,
And you have been trying with all your might,

Beware your possible fate,
You may be behind the "eight"—
You have probably gotten the shaft,
And brother, it's not fore, it's aft.

And finally,

What if Shakespeare Had Written

Shall I compare thee to a winter's night?
Thou art as cool and certainly as dark.
Howling winds give an October fright,
And winter's lease hath far too small a mark.
Sometime too cold the mouth of nature blows,
And often is her disposition chilled,
Upon a heart already deeply froze.
Should by chance nature's quest be unfulfilled?
But thy eternal winter shall not fade,
Nor lose possession of that cool thou owest,
Nor shall death brag thou in his bed be laid,
When in eternal rhymes to time thou goest.
So long as men can dream or wish for thee,
That long lives this and this says not to be.

One could speculate ad infinitum, some might infer ad nauseam (until sickness prevails), but the truth is, there is no end, the process regarding humor is as widespread as is our population.

On the other hand (I have five fingers), poetry can certainly be a healer. To the degree, that each of us is capable of delving into our innermost self, to that degree (using poetry) we can submit to the possibility that some good is obtained. To begin the process we only need to start writing about what we feel most strongly, beyond that, one can only guess.

There needs be no special structure; you build your poem the way you want. If a gift is evident, it cannot be hidden. I often think of what Emily Dickinson once said, *"If fame belonged to me, I could not escape her; if she did not, the longest day would pass me on the chase, and the approbation (warmly commending acceptance or agreement) of my dog would forsake(give up without a chance of return) me then."*

Using poetry to understand self a little better, is not a quest for fame, it is a look to understanding—a process of self-exploration using the coin of the realm, words. If nothing else, it will help a person better use the language of his inheritance; do we have another choice?

Certainly, we do if we speak more than one language. However, chances are your primary language will be your first choice. Nevertheless, for those who have a gift of another language, exploration will be even deeper, and the joy of discovery even more fruitful. After all, much of what poetry delivers to us has to do with sound. There you have it—Sound.

Going beyond words to sound is a way to place music to words. As you speak, your words in poetic form be aware that the sound is as important as the word. Your choice may indicate your way of relating to the world. However, the most important thing to remember is that you can do no wrong. No one can judge your work—you are the master of your creation, and the purpose here, is to create, nothing more, nothing less. There are ways to tune into your creative force.

Focus of the Senses,

An easy way to begin is to focus on past sensual stimulation to help you remember an event or feeling. The strongest sense is smell. The others in no particular order, sight, hearing and touch are important also. Often a triad of these senses will stimulate recall. When this happens, you can write about that experience. It may only be prose at first, but later form parts of what can be a poem. The important thing is that it produced recall—perhaps an event that is cause for consideration and perhaps healing. Many have spoken about getting something out of your system by restating what it means *today*. Often we find an old feeling has no validity *today*, what was once cause for concern is now a cause for laughter. Nuff said.

ENDNOTE 7

Communication

"Too often we underestimate the power of a touch, a smile, a kind word, a listening ear, an honest compliment, or the smallest act of caring, all of which have the potential to turn a life around."

—Leo Buscaglia

Communication Paradigm

Revisiting the concept of sense datum fixation will be necessary for this paradigm. The task of providing a systematic communication model for entry into another's body space will be the focus of this writing.

The three spaces are sight, voice and distant reduction zero, or contact space—which implies physical contact. Each space listed below given with a description of what to observe.

Sight Space—An observation of anyone coming into your sight space is usually in a perfunctory manner. Change the process to watchful waiting. Observe the posture, facies, and pace of movement, whether rapid or slow and notice if the person is looking at you or away. If the person is known, the process of reduction of distance between you will begin. If unknown, the process will be on hold until a signal by either person starts the reduction of distance between the two polarities i.e., unless they are just two ships passing in the night. Just joking.

Sight space entails all the surroundings. Therefore, depending on where you are will give you the necessary judgment to evaluate giving a sign for the person to come closer. The voice space is next.

Voice Space—The sound of the voice is a beginning for evaluation of the person's emotional state or well being. It is the primary step for evaluation of the words starting the conversation. I often remember the purr-words and snarl-words described by S.I. Hayakawa.[51] Voice sound will often give clue to one's feelings of the moment. In well-known personalities, evaluation may be easy. In unknown personalities, one should not guess but get feedback. With the completion of the first two spaces without conflict or a negative message, possible contact is imminent. This point reached, communication at a deeper level begins.

Distant Reduction Zero[52]—A kind of olfactory knowledge exists when *the contact space* is entered, in that; it is possible for one to process the expired microscopic droplets of another's system. Obviously, olfaction in the sense that one can recognize something of the immediate surroundings is common to all, but more importantly, an intimate relationship may exist with the process within the body chemistry. This may be so even without the person being aware of this relationship or even understanding one's feelings when such close contact exists.

---

[51] *Language in Thought and Action*, Hayakawa, S.I., Harcourt, Brace and Co., Inc., 1949, pg 44-46.
[52] Item reproduced from chapter five.

As primitive beings we relied on our olfactory ability to relieve our sexual tensions and today there can still be seen a strong vestigial response during courting behaviors. Each person is in touch with his surroundings with a special chemical space that is the byproducts of that person's metabolic state. It is the body's internal biorhythm sending signals resulting from the present state of feeling, health, or process of disease. If this is so, then a kind of chemical relationship exists within one's own bloodstream communicated to another by way of expired air from the sending system and is a situation that creates a kind of exocrine effect. This form of primal communication is not self evident for it is a process that we have long since forgotten how to recognize.

SENSE DATA RELATED TO[53]
STATES OF CONSCIOUSNESS

Senses	Conscious, Thinking	Subconscious or Preconscious	Unconscious
Sight	What is seen, the Actual reality as In looking at a picture Or landscape, however Much is left out due to Psychological selectivity.	That not seen by the The unaided eye, as In body aura, or Beyond the normal Color range.	Latent image, after Image as in photo- Graphic memory For some the ability To see an image of Things no longer in The present.
Hearing	The actual sound, as in voice, bell, or wind.	Beyond the range of Hearing as in dog whistle.	Sound of fear, sound Emanating from an Object that no one Else can hear, often A warning.

---

[53] Table reproduced from chapter six.

Smell	The actual smell, as in A banana, perfume, Food cooking, or for Some the ability to Process pheromone.	Memory recall, as in Bring one back in time. Some may be able to Decode the droplet Particles from another Body.	**Setting off the flight Or fight response Producing a panic Attack, pheromone Response.**
Taste	The actual taste, as in Food, banana, orange, Licorice or coffee.	When crossing over to Smell may bring back Old memories, but May be limited to Short-term memory.	**When crossing over To smell, may bring About similar Experience, but may Relate to long term Memory.**
Touch	The actual texture of an Object, thing or person, As well as temperature.	Latent qualities related To the objects Whereabouts, as in Being able to tell who Touched the object Last.	**Being able to pick up Qualities beyond the Here-and-now a Special knowledge About the person Who owned the Object as in persona, Good or bad karma.**

Passive imprints happen during stress. If a situation happens that provokes a strong emotional response, one may carry the baggage of that feeling around for many years. Posttraumatic stress disorder is probably a byproduct of such events. Passive imprints are not acquired with intent to remember, they are attached to strong stimuli that have driven a heavy nail into the brain. You cannot help but remember. Flashbacks happen when a present environment contains many of the sensual elements of the original event. At once, you are there again. When in contact with another's droplet space, a flashback may come from their being.

Flashbacks coming from processing another's neurochemical system differ from flashbacks of your own system. Your brain chemistry will decode the chemical message and attempt to put it in terms you can feel, see in your mind, or possibly hear in your mind. Nevertheless, there will be a change in your body chemistry noticeable to you. After close contact with another body system, it will take about 18-20 seconds for this process to begin. True communication at the microscopic level is never wrong, just very difficult to decipher. The best example is the one of sexual excitement. It is always quite understandable to men. However, decoding chemical messages having a different valence will require a different focus. Our perception of the chemical event made real by our ability to identify what the feelings mean to the other personality. This is no easy task and may take years to learn. Where verbal communication assists this process, is by using feedback. Especially, asking questions. A guide to this process is necessary.

The term thinking now added to the conscious block to indicate that this level requires conscious awareness. Awareness shall require being here now. This is a difficult process to learn. Intrusive thoughts not connected to the primary stimulus may cause one to lose focus. A guide to the process will help.

Sense Data Focus by Personality Dominance

Dominance	Situation	Sense
Psychointellectual When this part of the personality dominates the person's being intellectual pursuit is most evident.	According to what is being done. 1. Location, 2. Type of meeting, 3. Person known or not known, 4. Relationship with person, or 5. An unexpected occurrence.	Primary and level, as in taste, smell, etc. 1. Conscious, awareness of sense, as in smell, old memory recall.

		2. Preconscious, partial awareness of sense as in taste.
		3. Unconscious, reacting to an unknown sense stimulus.
Psychochemical Hedonism may be a prominent feature.	Contact 1. Handshake, 2. Massage, 3. Mucus contact, or 4. Sexual contact.	Example 1. Related to hand shake, touch. 2. Related to massage, touch. 3. As in kissing. 4. Sexual organ contact.
Psychespiritual Religiosity may prevail.	Primary 1. Usually as in praying. 2. All other aspects depend on the situation at hand, how one treats others and life decisions etc., one's moral code.	Example Living by the ten commandments or the golden rule, etc. The level may be conscious or unconscious. Sense of well being may not be ascribed to any one sense.

Depending on which part of the personality structure is dominant will fashion the behavior seen by others. Using the situation and the sense involvement shown in the forgoing gives a glimpse. If one is at distant reduction zero, touch—the processing of the expired droplets of another will cause a feeling. After 18-20 seconds, one must try to empty all intrusive thoughts and concentrate on being there, especially when it is another person. Often one is able to decipher the feelings with a mind picture, thought, or recognizable urge. The poem, taken from endnote 4, reduces the totality of sexual contact to orgasm.

Ecstasy

I like a look of passion
Because I know, it's true;
Men do not fake tumescence,
Nor simulate a semen flow.

The eyes with blank stare gaze,
And this is petit mort,
Impossible to sham;
Wet droplets upon the body clung,
By heated fervor flung.

Sweet daggers passion dipped,
Into entrails embedded,
Tasting nectar of love composed;
Two chemistries entwined,
Exploding, mixing timeless souls.

While not all contact between the sexes is sexual, it is a primary force, often influencing thought and action. Freud knew this, and it is probably why he gave emphasis to this part of the personality. While all communication between the male and female polarities has this root, a model for communication in general would benefit.

Walk Through Model for Distant Reduction Zero

Sight Space—Upon entering anyone's sight space take notice of all objects, happenings, and finally appearance of the person whose attention you want. If your gaze is not answered with some body movement or eye contact, reduce the space slightly. Once acknowledged, you may begin to reduce the distance between you. Continue your movement towards the person, being aware of any change that may signal alarm, as in, "go away."

Voice Space—At a comfortable distance use your voice; make the appropriate greeting for the circumstance. Listen for a response that allows further distance reduction. Listen for the growl or purr words. Pronunciation, word usage, vocabulary and rapidity of thought for all unknown personalities is important to evaluate. Evaluation will require more time and an environment conducive to talking. A place that allows for close contact without air draft is best for the contact space.

Contact Space—Depending on the situation, make the appropriate gesture of touch, as in, handshake, hug, etc. If the environment allows, wait 18-20 seconds for a feeling within, and takes into consideration that knowing at this time is important.

Summary from Earlier Chapter

Each person in your immediate environment has potential for giving you tension relief. Your polarity will be determined as you approach. Should this process produce encroachment upon another or feelings of uneasiness within yourself stop your approach and evaluate the situation. You might stop within the voice space and listen for a warning growl. Sometimes it has only been your speed of entry; trying to take up the distance too quickly.

You should experiment with the process of distant reduction with known personalities. Having some knowledge of their personality will help you with future evaluations when making contact with unknown personalities. Learn to read the *yes, yes* in her eyes and pheromones when her lips are saying *no, no*. Become familiar with those who light up when they see you. Be able to identify positive signals in distance reduction from those who send these signals to you most often.

Remember the three spaces: sight, voice, and contact. One must see you first, then one should hear the sound of your voice, and then contact may, or may not, be allowed. If allowed, try to focus on the chemical messages during the closeness by clearing your mind of all thoughts. Inhale the scent of the person and wait for 16-18 seconds for a new feeling within yourself. It will take much practice to learn how to evaluate the feelings.

A meaningful dialogue may be the result of a pleasurable contact after verbal communication has taken place. Moreover, it is *this* touch that feeds our soul, the act of human contact in a world of space, the temporary joining of separate nervous systems sharing a powerful nonverbal experience in the viscosity of time.

ENDNOTE 8

Mental Health

California Mental[54]
Health Is Going Down

They say mental health is going down,
Opinion, wide spread, mental health is dead.
Budget to smithereens been blown,
Patients from the coup been thrown;
Casualties from which the blood is bled.

They say our service is just a joke,
I'm sorry, sir, but the system's broke!
So when it's in a crisis you've been blown,
And it's to another door you've been shown,
You'll have to wait there until you croak.

They say mental health is about to fall,
I guess the message is finally known,
For those whose minds with sickness blown;
We're not our brothers' keeper, after all,
We're just here to watch him fall.

I have spent many years working within the mental health field. One of the best times that I can remember was working

---

[54]   *The Seduction of Time, et al,* Russell, Wm., Xlibris Corporation, 2004, pg 17.

at Comprehensive Mental Health in Tacoma, Washington, working as a member of the Community Support Team as a nurse counselor. During the years June 1981 to November 1986, I really believed that we were doing something to help the mentally ill. I have not seen such a team since.

I have been in Ukiah, California since November 1986. While I was acting as a Quality Assurance/ Utility Review Coordinator for Mendocino County Mental Health,[55] I often mentioned about getting a CST grant, and sadly to say, without results. Now retired, I am on the Mendocino County Mental Health Board, with the same impetus. My resolve is without change, and my results without success. Paperwork mounts high and meetings long, but little it seems to me, if anything, trickles down to the needy who wander the streets in mental quandaries. Communication complicated by many opinions, many thoughts, is a mental scrambled egg that defies separation. As always, with large committees, progress is sluggish at best. It is the old saying, many minds, and many opinions.

Legacy of the Damned[56]

Steeped in bureaucratic tripe
The mental health system dwells,
Sick itself, limping in the streets
        of uncertainty;
An amoeba-like entity that
Falls prey to any sweet seduction.

---

55   From 1986 to 1996.
56   Ibid., pg 23.

While agencies take their toll,
Like cancerous lesions that strangle
their host;
And everyone gets their monetary
share, save for the sick,
Who wander like zombies
in mental quandaries,
While paperwork mounts high,
A bloodless substitute for any cure,
And a monument to those who have
silently succumbed.

This is just a brief model of what the community support team should encompass. Today, 2014, the additional paperwork generated to apply for such a grant is almost prohibitive.

Community Support Teams
In Mental Health

Patients reside in our community. Some live in housing. Some live on the streets. However, they all live within our community. Often, when they decompensate, they require hospitalization. This costs money, money that most patients do not have. Yet, recidivism is the fact rather than the exception. Relapses occur often. For some, this is too often. The watchful eye of mental health technology has not been able to change the process. However, there have been some successful interventions by some clinics, not all in California, that have decreased the relapse time for some patients to the point that they could almost live "normal" lives. I know, some say that

1/3 of all schizophrenia cases will mend themselves. Yes and another 1/3 will be in and out of the hospital most of their lives, while a third 1/3 will be in the hospital most of their lives. With this knowledge, we should then change what we do. Some suggestions follow:

1. Probably with grant money, we should create teams of mental health workers. Perhaps we should start with just three teams. Each team would consist of a BA level counselor and a licensed psychiatric technician or a Licensed Vocational Nurse with a mental health background. A Licensed social worker should be the team leader. Each team would have sixty clients, thirty for each team member. The BA level worker would use the Licensed Vocational Nurse or Psych-Tech to assist with medication issues and shot clinics. Their primary responsibility would be to visit clients in their homes, or places where they reside. Weekly visits would be made during the intake period and continue until the client was stable.

2. The Licensed Certified Social Worker supervisor would only have a caseload of 15 clients. The primary duty of the supervisor would be to assist the teams with professional decisions regarding care and policy. Periodic meetings should take place where each team presents a case for discussion. Not only would this assist with helping the client, but it would also be a teaching tool for the team members. From a financial point of view, this would give the Community Support Teams the strength of seven (7) licensed social workers in essence, while only having one.

Obviously, the supervisor would also be doing chart review. Unless, of course, there was a Quality Assurance Nurse as part of the team.

3. A psychiatrist would be involved in all care. Each client is seen according to a schedule. It would be the duty of the Support Team Psych-Tech or Licensed Vocational Nurse to schedule the appointments with the psychiatrist. The Licensed Vocational Nurse (LVN) or Psych-Tech would sit in on the meeting with the psychiatrist unless the client objected. At that time, if the need for any long-term acting medicine, such as haldol or prolixin injection was necessary, the doctor would give the order and the LVN or Psych-Tech would administer the medication. Treatment plan review done as well.

4. Home visits and assistance with daily living is what is necessary to keep a client stable. If one monitors each client on a weekly basis, fewer chances for decompensation occur. The team members would be required to see clients as often as deemed necessary by the team's client review process. Assistance with daily activities can almost take any form of help; shopping for groceries, clothes, looking for a place to live et cetera.

5. Advocacy for the client is also necessary in care. If we do nothing else, we should be an advocate. Our community needs to know about mental illness. Our community needs to know what it can do to help. Without this knowledge, we stand helpless and watch our brother fail. Team effort

will be useless without the help the community can give. We need places for the homeless, the suffering and the impaired.

How can we have come this far without conquering mental illness is not the question? The question is. "How can we not commit ourselves to making a change?

You can find a more complete and up-to-date version on line, just type in team based services and you will appreciate why few even try for a grant.

In my opinion, it would be worth a try to pay someone with the expertise to write a grant, perhaps spending a little to get a lot.

ANNOTATED INDEX

CONTENTS

This is the acme of the hierarchy, the highest point of achievement in communication. Being fully achieved gives one the best chance of changing behavior in another. Changing behavior is what we do to survive. We change behavior of others on many levels, but written and verbal communication is the means for producing time gathering, the process that connects the past with the present. Connecting the past with the present should prevent us from repeating the same errors. It does not. This does not change the importance of this point once reached. An overall view of the communication process follows. 57

The forgoing written in 1976 at the time in my life that great change was happening. I was 43 years old. I was teaching in a military LPN (license vocational nurse) school. I had started teaching in September 1974. This then is the beginning of my self-realization, what my destiny was to become. Happenstance would have it that giving to others through teaching was my way of becoming. To ascend in any pillar one must have experience. Three faculties must exist to assist one in the climb to the acme of pillar success: 1. experience, 2. knowledge, and 3. health. In a way, they all exist together. Experience needs health and knowledge gained along the way. Knowledge is best gotten in a formal sense, which is, going to school or being in an apprenticeship. Vocational education may be best for many, as formal education often requires money and aptitude. Probably money is more often an obstacle than aptitude. Nevertheless, I have often assisted those who have less than the needed aptitude into finding their way to achieving a modicum of fulfillment in their chosen field. My gift may be to be able to assist one with their quest in a way that results in some kind of self-achievement. Instructors who are hypercritical and too full of themselves may emotionally cripple students. Every human being has worth; it is our duty to assist with finding a path to that worth. 97

After teaching for almost six years in the military LPN school,
I retired. As disheartening as this was, it was a necessary step. 98

DUTY TO SELF.. 99

After spending a very short time at Walla Walla State Penitentiary, in Walla Walla, Washington, and a couple of nursing care centers, I entered employment with Comprehensive Mental Health Center in Tacoma, Washington. As my resume reads, I had about 30 clients. This part of my experience, I am sure, gave me depth in understanding mental health disease as well as issues within the community. In fact, the experience assisted with my hire in my home state, California. After five years working with the mentally ill, I had a new outlook on life. Just having a degree in psychology does not give one experience; coming face-to-face with an ill mind, does............................. 99

I remember once when I was about five or so, I had an uncle that had a mural craft studio. He was a photographer back when photography was practically in its infancy. Well, perhaps not that far back, but it was about 1938 or so.

His laboratory was huge. There were large tanks and billboard type material strewn throughout this building. My cousin and I would play for hours in this vast place. Today the smell of hypo and developer still bring back those memories. The point in all of this is what he told me one day, "Billy my boy, when you grow up make your hobby your work, it is the best you can do. Do what you love." 99

Duty to self should be aimed at creating a hobby that can earn you a living. If not a hobby, then find something that you love and make that your life work. Either way you should enjoy what you do. Most often, when you are young it is not possible to do the forgoing. I wanted to be a chemist when I was young. I had a lab and spent many hours working on making explosives, and mixtures of chemicals in preparation for making rockets and the like. It was such fun. There was no pressure from anyone, and I could dream great dreams and build laboratories in the sky. Reality came crashing down when I entered junior college. Back in those days, 1953, they were using slide rules to do computation. Well, you guessed it, I was poor at learning this and the tedium leading into what I considered real chemistry was boring. The truth of the matter was that one must always start at the beginning, not in the middle. I was not mature enough at 20 to realize this, so I changed my major to psychology (sounds like a Freudian slip). After doing poorly with a grade point less than 2.0, I was drafted into the army. This was probably the best thing that could have happened, especially at the age of 21. 99

The problem with being in the army was that I had little time for duty to self. After two years spent mostly at Fort Ord, California, I received an honorable discharge, 100 dollars, and made the promise that I would join the active reserve unit in my hometown. This I did, at least for the first year. In 1957, I decided to go to Chico College, Chico California. I had been working in the PG&E office in my home town of Willits, California. I was a meter book clerk. This required a little math, legible printing, and taking in payments at the front counter. However, after about a year, I was finding the job pure drudgery, so I decided to go back to college. Off to Chico I went 100

College at the age of 24 would be a cinch, right! Wrong. I did not apply myself again, and after only one unsuccessful year and no improvement in grade point I dropped out, got married, and joined the army. This time I had a choice, so I enlisted with a preference in the medical field. After retaking a battery of tests, I had taken them before in 1954 as a draftee; my orders were to attend the Neuropsychiatry Basic Procedure Course given at Letterman

I was stationed at Fort Lewis, Washington assigned to the 47th Combat Support Hospital (MASH). My assignment to the 47th came right after I returned from Viet Nam in September of 1970. By 1974, I yearned to work again in the medical field proper; the 47th was primarily a training job with no exposure to real patients or hospital wards. To keep our proficiency within our military occupational specialty (MOS) we would rotate periodically working on a ward at Madigan Army Hospital. This was usually no longer than two or three months. Two or three months was not long enough to keep you up to date in your medical specialty, and you were lucky to get one rotation each year, usually around the time that you were required to take your yearly proficiency test. The powers-that-be did not want their clinical specialists to do poorly on the test. Besides that, if you did not do well you would lose your $75.00 proficiency pay. It was time for me to look for a better assignment. 103

I found out that there was an opening at the advanced medical specialist school Madigan Army Medical Center. I put in the paperwork and on September 2, 1974, I reported to my new duty station. However, I had to attend an Administrative Faculty Development Course given at the Academy of Health Science at Fort Sam Houston, Texas and take the Washington state test for licensed practical nurses before I would be a fully accredited instructor. By the end of 1974, I was ready to start the job of teaching at the Patient Care Specialist Course, Madigan Army Medical Center Tacoma, Washington. However, the journey had just begun. Every journey begins with a first step, as an instructor, that first step is the preparation of behavioral objectives, the DNA of your lesson plan. 103

Having just recently graduated from a faculty development course, I was acutely aware of the need to make instruction meaningful, concise, and testable. One method that was in vogue regarded the practice of using instructional objectives from a book by Robert F. Mager. The key word in all of this is testable. 104

In order for anything to be testable, the instructional objectives should follow a threefold presentation: 104

1. Performance. An objective always says what a learner is expected to be able to do; the objective sometimes describes the outcome, the product or result of the doing (behavior) 104

2. Condition. An objective always describes the important conditions under which the performance (behavior) is to occur. 104

3. Criterion. Wherever possible, an objective describes the criterion of acceptable performance by describing how well the learner must perform in order to be considered acceptable, often describing the minimum acceptable behavior or performance. This threshold allows for assigning a grade in most cases.. 104

Ideally, you would also have a manuscript of the complete instruction, word for word. In the event that you were unable to teach a class, another could do so with the help of the lesson plan and manuscript. I do not know any instructors (today) that have a manuscript. Most instructors just have good notes written on their lesson plan. I have only one such manuscript made when I was attending the faculty development school. I do however have some damn good lesson plans. If you know your subject, you will only need a good lesson plan..106

In the six years of teaching within the military clinical specialist course, I grew exponentially as a soldier, as an instructor, and as a person. However, by 1980 I was ready for the next step, returning to civilian life. After 24 years in the military with 1 year in Vietnam and 3 years in Japan, I was ready to find a place and put down some roots. My last year teaching would probably not have been my last year in the army if I had not gotten orders for Germany. After trying to get a relief from orders with no success, I decided that retirement was my best option. In June 1980, I took terminal leave, and finally, said goodbye to a place in life that I shall always miss.............. 106

This, however, is not the end of the story. I was 47 with a realization that teaching was my place, my destination, and my resolve; finally, I had arrived. There was still much to learn, but I had been given the opportunity to experience a great deal up to this point. I was honorably discharged into civilian life..107

Finding a job teaching so soon after leaving the service was unlikely, but I needed to do something, I was too young to retire fulltime. There were short-term jobs, mostly working with nursing care facilities and mental health services. Finally, I got a job working with a mental health clinic, Comprehensive Mental Health Center, Tacoma, Washington. It was a good job with a great deal to be learned and done. After about two years, I began teaching at a business school in the evening while continuing to work at my day job. I often spent 14 or more hours working each day. The important part of this was that I again taught medical terminology, a subject that I had taught in the military. This time, however, I used a text supplied by the school. In the earlier years, teaching in the military we just put together a course using the books available aided by a good lesson plan. This was mostly just a memorization process often quite difficult for students. The course at the business school consisted of a filmstrip with audio and a book to follow. My primary duty was one of giving the required tests. Any questions from the students were squeezed in at the end of the filmstrip lesson. Not the ideal way to teach even though the author of the book claimed that the average grade for students taking this course was 90 plus percent. As doubtful as I thought that was, I made no changes, nor did I suggest any to the powers-that-be. The students taking the course that I guided averaged about 80 plus percent. It would be much later that I would develop a course of my own, similar but in no way congruent. 107

Coming Full Circle.. 108

It should be the responsibility of anyone having the duty to teach to be aware of his or her motivation, need, desire, or reason for doing so. A firm platform of conviction may not be enough. Each of us has an internal vision of how we think the world is. Having an awareness of that internal view and the way it fits with the true reality of existence gives one a beginning for the quest for truth. How one lives one's life, is as important as what one believes, for the two are often inseparable (At this point my personal creed is inserted, page   ) 128

In the late summer of 2006, I was informed that my medical terminology class would be changed to a distant learning style. I was also told that eventually my class would become an online course. I thought that I would try the online course when it came time, hoping that it would be several years before that happened..128

While teaching my last regular class in the fall of 2006, I began filming the part of the class that used flashcards based on the book, Medical Terminology by the Mnemonic Story System. I did the filming during an actual class. I also had given to the dean of instruction a well-written lesson plan describing the preparation for the class. This plan was both a description and a permission to do. The following spring the first class began. The following is the syllabus used for the class. 128

Communication and Living   293

One of the reasons that I decided that changing to an online course was a poor idea had to do with the faltering condition of the distant learning course I was teaching. In the past, for each semester, I would write a summary of the course for the powers-that-be. It was obvious to me that the distant learning course I was presently teaching, in preparation to an online course, had its share of shortcomings. I had put hours of work into the course, CD creation, my book, and a complete syllabus, shown earlier. However, it was not enough. Although the following summary is without negative comments by the students, it does not give a good evaluation when you compare it with past classes..220

There is a ubiquitous cloud that is about to befall us. No one seems to care. Learning is about to be dealt a blow so severe that all but a few classrooms will be left. This oncoming tidal wave is in the form of online education; a bloodless form of learning so simplistically seductive that the danger remains hidden from view..228

With our present education system, wallowing in the mud of imperfection, the chosen way of least resistance is online teaching. The classroom size will dwindle until only the powerful computer shall stand, cold, bloodless, and impervious to human thought or question. We need to get back to some of the ways of yesteryear, a philosophical backward glance of the not too long ago.

Sometime in 1976, I wrote what I called then, My Personal Creed. Over the years, it has been revisited by many different names: A Nurses Prayer, A Mantra for Living to name a few (Chapter 9).

The creed now updated, with paragraph 6, a place with four corners called a room.

6. Give me a place where I can touch the lives of those in quest of knowledge with communication. A place with four corners called a room. Learning should take place with a breathing, feeling person that can provide feedback; let me be that someone. Human thought is done best when shared with another face to face.

www.ingramcontent.com/pod-product-compliance
Lightning Source LLC
Chambersburg PA
CBHW020731180526
45163CB00001B/193